Pediatric Headaches
in Clinical Practice

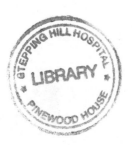

Pediatric Headaches
in Clinical Practice

Andrew D. Hershey, MD, PhD, FAHS

Cincinnati Children's Hospital Medical Center, Professor of Pediatrics and Neurology University of Cincinnati, College of Medicine, Cincinnati, OH, USA

Scott W. Powers, PhD, ABPP, FAHS

Cincinnati Children's Hospital Medical Center, Professor of Pediatrics Division of Behavioral Medicine and Clinical Psychology University of Cincinnati, College of Medicine Cincinnati, OH, USA

Paul Winner, DO, FAAN, FAAP, FAHS

Palm Beach Neurology, West Palm Beach, FL, Clinical Professor of Neurology Nova Southeastern University, Fort Lauderdale, FL USA

Marielle A. Kabbouche, MD

Cincinnati Children's Hospital Medical Center, Assistant Professor of Pediatrics and Neurology, University of Cincinnati, College of Medicine, Cincinnati, OH, USA

WILEY-BLACKWELL

A John Wiley & Sons, Ltd., Publication

This edition first published 2009, © 2009 John Wiley & Sons, Ltd

Wiley-Blackwell is an imprint of John Wiley & Sons, formed by the merger of Wiley's global Scientific, Technical and Medical business with Blackwell Publishing.

Registered office: John Wiley & Sons Ltd, The Atrium, Southern Gate, Chichester, West Sussex, PO19 8SQ, UK

Other Editorial Offices:
9600 Garsington Road, Oxford, OX4 2DQ, UK
111 River Street, Hoboken, NJ 07030-5774, USA

For details of our global editorial offices, for customer services and for information about how to apply for permission to reuse the copyright material in this book please see our website at www.wiley.com/wiley-blackwell

The right of the author to be identified as the author of this work has been asserted in accordance with the Copyright, Designs and Patents Act 1988.

Wiley also publishes its books in a variety of electronic formats. Some content that appears in print may not be available in electronic books.

Designations used by companies to distinguish their products are often claimed as trademarks. All brand names and product names used in this book are trade names, service marks, trademarks or registered trademarks of their respective owners. The publisher is not associated with any product or vendor mentioned in this book. This publication is designed to provide accurate and authoritative information in regard to the subject matter covered. It is sold on the understanding that the publisher is not engaged in rendering professional services. If professional advice or other expert assistance is required, the services of a competent professional should be sought.

The contents of this work are intended to further general scientific research, understanding, and discussion only and are not intended and should not be relied upon as recommending or promoting a specific method, diagnosis, or treatment by physicians for any particular patient. The publisher and the author make no representations or warranties with respect to the accuracy or completeness of the contents of this work and specifically disclaim all warranties, including without limitation any implied warranties of fitness for a particular purpose. In view of ongoing research, equipment modifications, changes in governmental regulations, and the constant flow of information relating to the use of medicines, equipment, and devices, the reader is urged to review and evaluate the information provided in the package insert or instructions for each medicine, equipment, or device for, among other things, any changes in the instructions or indication of usage and for added warnings and precautions. Readers should consult with a specialist where appropriate. The fact that an organization or Website is referred to in this work as a citation and/or a potential source of further information does not mean that the author or the publisher endorses the information the organization or Website may provide or recommendations it may make. Further, readers should be aware that Internet Websites listed in this work may have changed or disappeared between when this work was written and when it is read. No warranty may be created or extended by any promotional statements for this work. Neither the publisher nor the author shall be liable for any damages arising herefrom.

Library of Congress Cataloguing-in-Publication Data

Pediatric headaches in clinical practice / Andrew D. Hershey ... [et al.].
   p. ; cm.
  Includes bibliographical references and index.
  ISBN 978-0-470-51273-9 (cloth)
  1. Headache in children. I. Hershey, Andrew D.
  [DNLM: 1. Headache Disorders. 2. Adolescent. 3. Child. 4. Headache.
  5. Pediatrics–methods. WL 344 P371 2009]
  RJ496.H3P33 2009
  618.92'8491–dc22

                                2008053890

ISBN: 9780470512739

A catalogue record for this book is available from the British Library.

Typeset in 10.5/13pt Times by Thomson Digital, Noida, India.
Printed in Singapore by Markono Print Media Pte Ltd.

First Impression 2009

Contents

Preface

Head pain is a nearly universal experience for humans, yet it remains poorly recognized as a significant problem. The experience has been observed across all ages, yet the presentation and underlying etiology vary across the developmental scale. In the developing nervous system, these changes occur rapidly as a child's awareness and ability to express this symptom as a problem mature and the very nature of the symptoms evolves. Although many of the well observed patterns of adult head pain are applicable to children, the unique aspects of evaluating and treating children in association with the variations that occur in childhood headache disorders continue to make the management of these diseases a challenge. A perspective that goes beyond the downward application of information derived from the adult headache experience is needed. This book will help you answer challenges specific to pediatric headache.

This universal nature of head pain creates a familiarity that is both a barrier and a challenge. Too often, pain has been ignored as a legitimate or serious condition, and care has relied on experience and anecdotal reasoning that many times have proven false. As scientific understanding has progressed to the recognition that head pain is a component of a disease process with a vast range of underlying disorders and presentations, new advances have begun to be applied. Recognition of the symptom as only one component of a disease process has lead to many of the recent discoveries underlying the improved diagnosis and treatment of both primary and secondary disorders.

This book describes how to apply the present scientific advances to the clinical practice of headache medicine in children and adolescents. Future advances will help to refine our abilities to reduce the burden and disability due to headaches for children as they mature into adulthood. By combining our clinical and research experience in childhood headache medicine, we aim to help you deliver the latest advances in the management of childhood headaches.

Andrew D. Hershey
Scott W. Powers
Paul Winner
Marielle A. Kabbouche

1

History of childhood headaches

Andrew D. Hershey

Headaches in children, adolescents and adults are quite common. The study and characterization of childhood headaches, however, entered an era of increased interest with the adoption of the first edition of the *International Classification of Headache Disorders* [1].

The initial description of headaches in humans is quite old. Ancient writings in an epic poem from the Sumerian area dating back to 3000 BC describe what appear to be migraine-type headaches (i.e. 'the sick headache').

> The sick-eyed says not
> "I am sick-eyed"
> The sick-headed not
> "I am sick-headed" [2]

The oldest known medical manuscript, a 3500-year-old papyrus found in the tomb of Thebes and translated by George Ebers in 1874 refers to 'a sickness of half the head' [3].

From the Mesopotamian literature, a migraine with aura appears to be described as: 'the head is bent with pain gripping his temples' and 'a man's brain contains fire and myalgia afflicts the temples and smites the eyes, his eyes are afflicted with dimness and cloudiness' [4, 5]. Hippocrates in approximately 400 BC also described what appears to be a migraine with aura that was relieved by emesis as 'a shining light ... followed by violent pain beginning in the temples and eventually reaching the entire head and neck area' [6–9].

Pediatric Headaches in Clinical Practice   Andrew D. Hershey, Paul Winner, Marielle A. Kabbouche and Scott W. Powers
© 2009 John Wiley & Sons, Ltd.

The specific discoverer of migraine, however, is often credited as Aretaeus of Cappadocia in the second century [10]. He described a mild, infrequent headache lasting a few days – cephalagia (i.e. tension headache); a longer, more severe and less responsive headache – cephalia; and a one-sided headache with blackness before the eyes, nausea, vomiting, photophobia and osmophobia – heterocrania (i.e. migraine) [11, 12]. For the heterocrania he described a 6–24 h headache that could be on either side, front or vertical [12].

The term migraine (from the Greek *hemicrania*) appears to have been first introduced by Galen in the second century [3]. He described 'Hemicrania is a painful disorder affecting approximately one half of the head, either the right or the left side, and which extends along the length of the longitudinal suture . . . . It is caused by the ascent of vapours, either excessive in amount, or too hot, or too cold'.

The study of headaches from a modern, scientific point of view began in the 1700s. Tissot attempted to differentiate migraines from other headaches by describing them as a neuralgia provoked by reflexes from the stomach, gall bladder or uterus [4, 13]. Fotherfill in 1778 provided a detailed description of a migraine attack is his paper 'Remarks on the complaint commonly known under the name of the Sick Headache' [3]. In 1873, Liveing gave a detailed description of megrim or sick headaches [14]. Many of the features he described in that paper continue to be recognized as clinical features today for migraine headaches.

1.1 Childhood headaches

Headaches in adults have been examined by many well-known neurologists. In children, however, the historical study of headache is much more limited. Tissot [13], Calmeil [15] and Living [14] referred to childhood headaches in their discussion of migraines [4]. This was limited to the observation that migraines may start in childhood. The initial description of childhood headaches themselves began to appear in the early 1900s [16–20]. These papers began to identify that children could suffer from the same headache disorders as adults, but with subtle variations.

One of the early theories on childhood migraines, as well as some adult migraines, was the possible causal relationship to allergy. Balyeat and Rinkel [18] in 1931 reported on their experience with migraine. They noted that 30% of their patients developed their symptoms before 10 years old. They related migraine to allergy based on the observation that many of the very young children came in with a complaint of allergies, but historical review revealed the presence of migraines. They also drew this conclusion based on the persistent family history of allergies and the presence of 'food allergies' (i.e. food triggers) presenting as cyclic vomiting. Ogden [21] in 1961, upon reviewing his studies, concluded that migraine and allergy may very well be related, but could not clearly define how. Stevenson [22] compiled much of this information in 1993 and concluded that the high frequency of both disorders contributed to this apparent relationship.

In 1949, Vahlquist and Hackzell [23] began a much more extensive study of childhood headaches. They reported their findings on 31 patients with onset of headache between age 1 and 4 years. This paper described patients that they had identified with migraine headaches. In doing so they began to develop criteria by which childhood migraines could be diagnosed. In contrast to the observations in adults, their study they noted a predominance of males [23], that children may have short-duration headaches, temperature may change during a headache, a psychogenic element is very important, and allergies or food sensitivities do not always bear out. One of the most significant features of this study and subsequent work was the initial establishment of criteria for the diagnosis of childhood headaches. These criteria described paroxysmal headaches that included two of four features: a pain occurring in only part of the head, the presence of nausea, the presence of a flimmer scotoma and a positive family history. Although these features do not meet the current criteria for diagnosis of migraines in adults or children, they did provide an initial framework for the study of childhood headaches. In 1955, Vahlquist in collaboration with Bille, Ekstrand and Hackzell used these initial criteria to screen 1236 school children between the ages of 10 and 12 years old for the presence of migraines [4]. They found the prevalence of migraines was 4.5%, while the prevalence of nonmigrainous headaches was 13.3%.

During the 1950s, several groups reported on their experience with childhood migraines and the features that may differentiate them from the adult migraine patients. Micheal and Williams [24] remarked in the 20 patients they followed that there was a significant association with seizure disorders. Krupp and Friedman [25] found that a large fraction of the 600 adults they studied had the onset of their migraines in childhood. They went on to characterize 50 children with migraines, finding that the headaches were quite similar to the adults they studied. The exceptions they noted were that these headaches were milder and had more significant gastrointestinal and psychological aspects. Glaser [26] reported his observations in 1954. He focused on the allergic component of childhood headaches, but did not conclude that there was a need to test for food allergies. He also noted that the onset may occur as early as infancy. In 1956, Burke and Peters [27] reported on their 6-year study of 92 patients, noting a higher incidence of migraines in childhood headaches than previously reported and a positive treatment response to aspirin, ergotamine/ caffeine, and diphenylhydantoin.

In 1962, Bille [4] expanded on this study in his very thorough work on headache in children. In the preface to this study, he discussed several historical observations about childhood headaches. These included that childhood attacks are more frequent, have a shorter duration with a shorter prodrome and have scotomas less frequently. In addition, the headache attacks appear to be less severe, have predominance of gastrointestinal symptoms, including cyclic vomiting and attacks of abdominal pain, and high fevers may be associated with headaches.

In Bille's study, he provided questionnaires to 9059 school children in Uppsala, Sweden, aged 7–15 years old attending school in 1955. It excluded children with mental handicaps or those who were attending vocational schools. The children and their parents were asked about the presence of headaches and, if headaches were present, they were asked to describe the features of the headaches. He received 8993 replies (99.3%). The children were then divided into four groups: (1) children who never had a headache – 3720 (41.1%); (2) children with rare nonparoxysmal headaches – 4316 (48.0%); (3) children with frequent nonparoxysmal headaches – 473 (5.3%); and (4) children with paroxysmal headaches – 484 (5.4%). He felt the last group represented the children with migraines. In this group, in addition to the headache being paroxysmal, he reported the most frequently cited features of these headaches were one-sided pain, nausea, visual aura, and a positive family history. From this study, he identified that approximately 25% of children reported a significant headache by age 5 years and that 75% of children had reported a significant headache by age 15 years. Within this age range they were able to suggest a frequency range for migraines from 1 to 7% dependent on age and sex. To assess the headache diagnosis more accurately, he contacted every fifth child in the 'migraine' group and every tenth child in the non-migrainous paroxysmal group. He was then able to estimate the frequency of migraine to be 3.97% (357 out of 8993). He also characterized the lack of differences in these children compared with their headache-free counterparts in school performance, school attendance, or socioeconomics status. He further described the characteristics of these children and their headaches, including detailed features of the headaches, pediatric and neurological examinations, and electroencephalogram (EEG) examination. He has subsequently followed 73 children in the migraine group for up to 40 years [28]. Of these adults, 23% were migraine free by age 25 years; however, more than half continued to have migraines at age 50 years.

In 1976, Sillanpää [29] performed a similar study to Bille's. His study differed in that he questioned 4825 children aged 7 years old and found a prevalence of migraines at this age of 3.9%. He used the Vahlquist criteria for the diagnosis of migraines and found that 37% of the children reported a headache of any type. In 1983, he described the results of a 7-year follow-up on 2915 of these children [30]. He found that in those 7 years the prevalence of headaches increased to 69% and the prevalence of migraines increased to 6.6% with the greatest increase occurring in girls (14.8%). He also noted that this appeared to be a continuous trend of increasing frequency as the children advanced through adolescence.

In 1976, Prensky [31] reviewed the differences in children's migraines versus adult migraine. Some of the differences that he noted between children and adults were that there was a slight predominance of males (~60% versus ~33%), less likelihood of unilateral headache (25–66% versus 75–91%), more nausea/vomiting (70–100% versus 60–90%), less visual aura (10–50% versus 60–75%), and an increased incidence of seizures (5.4–12.3% versus <3%). He also noted that the familial incidence was approximately the same (72% versus 71%).

In 1984, Barlow [32] published his book giving a descriptive account on childhood migraines. Much of this information is based on personal observations on 300 children with headaches over a 20-year period. Through these observations, as well as a review of the literature, he focused on his experience with managing childhood headaches and the problems that arise. This included not only migraines, but also migraine variants, the periodic syndrome, psychogenic headaches, traumatic headaches, symptomatic headaches, and various treatment designs.

In 1994, Abu-Arefeh and Russell [33] reported a similar study to Bille's of 1962 using the International Headache Society (IHS) criteria. By using these criteria they identified that approximately 10.2% of children between the ages of 5 and 15 years met the IHS criteria for migraine headaches. Whether this implies a trend of an increasing frequency of migraine headaches or whether the use of the IHS criteria provides for more specific identification is unclear. However, the authors feel that the most likely explanation is the increasing frequency of headaches within a population. This is mirrored by studies in adults that agree with the increasing trend of the frequency of headaches.

1.2 Migraine variants and the periodic syndromes

A unique feature in the childhood headache and migraine spectrum that has historically been noted is often referred to as periodic syndromes of childhood or migraine variants. Wyllie and Schlesinger described the periodic syndrome as having a combination of symptoms [34, 35], including one or more of:

1. cyclic vomiting of repeated bilious attacks;

2. recurrent vague abdominal complaints;

3. recurrent headaches;

4. dizzy spells;

5. periodic attacks of fever;

6. periodic attacks of limb and joint pains or stiffness.

In Prensky's review of migraine variants [31], he referred to these migraine variants as a 'recurrent syndrome'. He described this syndrome as 'recurrent abdominal pain with or without nausea and vomiting, cyclic vomiting, associated fever, and autonomic symptoms such as pallor and sweating as well as chest pains and leg cramps'. He reviewed 11 published series of such children, and although finding that 43% of these children had recurrent headaches, there were notable differences with the migraine group (less commonly male, more frequent seizures and paroxysmal discharges on EEG, more frequent history of seizures and less frequent history of migraines).

In Barlow's chapter on the periodic syndrome [32], he referred to Cullen and MacDonald's [36] conclusion that 'juvenile migraine is another nave for "periodic syndrome"'. He went on to review the literature and focus further on his experience with cyclic vomiting/recurrent episodic vomiting and 'abdominal migraine'/paroxysmal abdominal pain. He discussed several migraine variants that he had seen (including fever with migraine, paroxysmal leg pain and paroxysmal chest pain) that may be considered part of migraine variants or the periodic syndrome.

Other childhood variants of migraines have also been described. One of these is benign paroxysmal vertigo of childhood. Basser [37] originally described this in 1964 and Fenichel [38] related migraine as a cause for this in 1967. In a recent long-term follow-up, Lindskog *et al.* [39] reported that 13–20 years after the diagnosis of benign paroxysmal vertigo of childhood they were able to conclude that it is a benign illness that migraine may cause, but that migraine is not a general precursor.

In 1969, Snyder [40] described a disorder of recurrent torticollis in infancy. Its exact etiology is unknown. Deonna [41] reviewed the possible association of this entity with migraines with the conclusion that so few patients have been accurately recorded that a direct relationship with migraine, although it may be possible, cannot be made for certain.

Another group of variants that have been described in children has been reviewed by Hosking [42] in which there is an alteration of consciousness or interaction with their environment. These include confusional migraine, the Alice in Wonderland syndrome, migraine stupor and transient global amnesia. Many of these unusual symptoms were described in children in the 1970s by various authors and are important to differentiate from other causes of acute alterations in consciousness.

1.3 Classification and criteria for headaches

Historically, the criteria for the diagnosis of childhood headache disorders relied predominantly on the clinician's impression. The Vahlquist criteria discussed above began to provide a basis by which childhood headaches could be studied and remained the central criteria for the study of childhood headaches and migraines. These criteria focused on the paroxysmal nature of migraine headaches in children with a few selective features (two of four features: a pain occurring in only part of the head, the presence of nausea, the presence of a flimmer scotoma and a positive family history).

During the same time period that Vahlquist and Bille were beginning to describe and classify childhood headaches, the Ad Hoc Committee on Classification of Headache suggested a classification scheme for headaches in adults [43]. This 1962 commentary suggested 15 different headache classifications, including 'vascular headache of migraine type', 'muscle-contraction headache' and 'combined headache'. Although this classification scheme differentiated headache types, it did not provide specific criteria for individual headache subtypes.

In 1979, Prensky and Sommer [44], based on a retrospective study of 84 children that had been clinically defined as having migraines, suggested refining the criteria for childhood headaches. Their criteria were:

1. recurrent headaches with symptom-free intervals;

2. three of six symptoms:

    (a) abdominal pain, nausea or vomiting with the headache;

(b) hemicrania;

(c) a throbbing, pulsatile quality of pain;

(d) complete relief after a brief period of rest;

(e) an aura, either visual, sensory or motor;

(f) a history of migraine headaches in one of more members of the immediate family.

In addition, they found 17 had paroxysmal discharges on EEG, a slight predominance of males (especially in children under 11 years), a predominant frontal location to the headache, and that about one-half of the children had a 50% reduction in their headache frequency independent of the treatment 6 months following a neurologist visit.

Although others have also suggested childhood headache criteria [45–48], no standardized criteria had been established. This left much of the reported studies of headaches, both in children and adults, to be based on an individual clinician's clinical diagnosis of headaches and migraines. In 1988, the IHS provided a major advancement in the further study of headaches when it published its initial IHS criteria. These criteria were developed by multiple headache researchers and used both clinical opinions and reported character-izations of individual headache types. In these criteria they established 12 different major headache types that could be roughly divided into primary headaches and secondary headaches. This work delineated detailed criteria for all headache types. These criteria also serve as the basis for the modern study of headaches in adults and children, with many of the observations and studies discussed throughout the remainder of the book using these criteria as a foundation for the scientific study of headache. The future will hold many new advances and discoveries for the treatment of childhood headaches are there, and the remaining chapters of this book will delineate our current understanding of childhood headaches.

References

1. Headache Classification Committee of the International Headache Society (1988) Classification and diagnostic criteria for headache disorders, cranial neuralgias and facial pain. *Cephalalgia: An International Journal of Headache,* **8**(S7), 1–96.
2. Alvarez, W. (1945) Was there sick headache in 3000 B.C.? *Gastroenterology,* **5**, 524.
3. Hanington, E. (1973) *Migraine,* Priory Press Limited, London.

4. Bille, B.S. (1962) Migraine in school children. A study of the incidence and short-term prognosis, and a clinical, psychological and electroencephalographic comparison between children with migraine and matched controls. *Acta Paediatrica (Oslo, Norway: 1992) Supplement*, **136**, 1–151.

5. Sigerist, H.E. (1951) *A History of Medicine. Volume 1: Primitive and Archaic Medicine*, Oxford University Press, New York, NY.

6. Silberstein, S.D., Lipton, R.B. and Goadsby, P.J. (1998) *Headache in Clinical Practice*, Isis Medical Media, Ltd, Oxford, UK.

7. Plato (1960) The Republic, in *The Collected Dialogues of Plato* (eds E. Hamilton and H. Cairns), Pantheon Books, New York, p. 103.

8. Lance, J.W. (1982) *Mechanism and Management of Headache*, 4th edn, Butterworth Scientific, London.

9. Edmeads, J. (1990) The treatment of headache: a historical perspective, in *Drug Therapy for Headache* (ed. R.M. Gallagher), Marcel Dekker, Inc., New York, pp. 1–8.

10. Waters, W.E. (1986) *Headache*, Series in Clinical Epidemiology, PSG Publishing Company, Inc., Littleton, MA.

11. Critchley, M. (1967) Migraine: from Cappadocia to Queen Square, in *Background to Migraine: First Migraine Symposium* (ed. R. Smith), Heinemann, London, pp. 22–38.

12. Rose, F.C. (1995) The history of migraine from Mesopotamian to Medieval times. *Cephalalgia: An International Journal of Headache*, **S15**, 1–3.

13. Tissot, S.-A. (1783) Traité des nerfs et de leurs maladies. De le catalepsie, de l'exstase, de l'andesthésie de la migraine et des maladies du cerveau, in *Oeuvres de Monsieur Tissot*, P. F. Didot le jeune, Paris.

14. Liveing, E. (1873) *On Megrim, Sick-Headache, and Some Allied Disorders: A Contribution to the Pathology of Nerve-Storms*, J. and A. Churchill, London.

15. Calmeil, H. (1832–1846) Migraine, in *Dictionnaire de Médecine* (ed. N.P. Adelon), Béchet jeune, Paris.

16. Comby, J. (1921) La migraine chez les enfants. *Arch de Médec des Enfants*, **24**, 29–49.

17. Curschmann, H., (1922) ber Kindemigräne. *Münchener Medizinische Wochenschrift*, **69**, 1746.

18. Balyeat, R.M. and Rinkel, H.J. (1931) Allergic migraine in children. *American Journal of Diseases of Children*, **42**, 1126–1133.

19. Debre, R. and Broca, R. (1935) La migraine chez l'enfant et son équivalent abdominal. *Le Bulletin Medical*, **49**, 467–477.

20. Riley, H.A., (1937) Migraine in children and the mechanism of the attack. *Bulletin of the Neurological Institute of New York*, **6**, 387.

21. Ogden, H.D. (1961) The relationship of allergy to headache. *Headache*, **1**, 14–19.

22. Stevenson, D.D. (1993) Allergy, atopy, nasal disease, and headache, in *Wolff's Headache and Other Head Pain*, 6th edn (eds D.J. Dalessio and S.D. Siberstein), Oxford University Press, Oxford, pp. 291–333.

23. Vahlquist, B. and Hackzell, G. (1949) Migraine of early onset. A study of thirty one cases in which the disease first appeared between one and four years of age. *Acta Paediatrica*, **38**, 622–636.

24. Micheal, M.I. and Williams, J.M. (1952) Migraine in children. *The Journal of Pediatrics*, **41**, 18–24.

25. Krupp, G.R. and Friedman, A.P. (1953) Migraine in children. *American Journal of Diseases of Children*, **85**, 146–150.

26. Glaser, J. (1954) Migraine in pediatric practice: observations with special reference to migraine of allergic origin. *American Journal of Diseases of Children*, **88**, 92–98.

27. Burke, E.C. and Peters, G.A. (1956) Migraine in childhood: a preliminary report. *American Journal of Diseases of Children*, **92**, 330–336.

28. Bille, B. (1997) A 40-year follow-up of school children with migraine. *Cephalalgia: An International Journal of Headache*, **17**, 488–491.

29. Sillanpää, M. (1976) Prevalence of migraine and other headache in Finnish children starting school. *Headache*, **15**, 288–290.

30. Sillanpää, M. (1983) Changes in the prevalence of migraine and other headaches during the first seven school years. *Headache*, **23**, 15–19.

31. Prensky, A.L. (1976) Migraine and migrainous variants in pediatric patients. *Pediatric Clinics of North America*, **23**(3), 461–471.

32. Barlow, C.F. (1984) *Headaches and Migraine in Childhood*, Spastics International Medical Publications, London.

33. Abu-Arafeh, I. and Russell, G. (1994) Prevalence of headache and migraine in school-children. *British Medical Journal*, **309**, 765–769.

34. Wyllie, W.G. and Schlesinger, B., (1933) The periodic group of disorders in childhood. *British Journal of Children's Diseases*, **30**, 349–351.

35. Silberstein, S.D. and Saper, J.R. (1993) Migraine: diagnosis and treatment, in *Wolff's Headache and Other Head Pain*, 6th edn, (eds D.J. Dalessio and S.D. Siberstein), Oxford University Press, Oxford, pp. 96–170.

36. Cullen, K.J. and MacDonald, W.B. (1963) The periodic syndrome: it's nature and prevalence. *Medical Journal of Australia*, **50**, 167–173.

37. Basser, L.S. (1964) Benign paroxysmal vertigo of childhood. *Brain: A Journal of Neurology*, **87**, 141–152.

38. Fenichel, G.M. (1967) Migraine as a cause of benign paroxysmal vertigo of childhood. *The Journal of Pediatrics*, **71**, 114–115.

39. Lindskog, U., Odkvist, L., Noaksson, L. and Wallquist, J. (1999) Benign paroxysmal vertigo in childhood: a long-term follow-up. *Headache*, **39**, 33–37.

40. Snyder, C.H. (1969) Paroxysmal torticollis in infancy: a possible form of labyrinthitis. *American Journal of Diseases of Children*, **117**, 458–460.

41. Deonna, T.W. (1988) Paroxysmal disorders which may be migraine or may be confused with it, in *Migraine in Childhood* (ed. J.M. Hockaday), Butterworths, London, pp. 75–87.

42. Hosking, G. (1988) Special forms: variants of migraine in childhood, in *Migraine in Childhood*, (ed. J.M. Hockaday), Butterworths, London, pp. 35–53.

43. Friedman, A.P., Finley, K.H. *et al.* (1962) Classification of headache: Ad Hoc Committee on Classification of Headache. *The Journal of the American Medical Association*, **179**(9), 127–128.

44. Prensky, A.L. and Sommer, D. (1979) Diagnosis and treatment of migraine in children. *Neurology*, **29**, 506–510.

45. Deubner, D.C. (1977) An epidemiologic study of migraine and headache in 10–20 year olds. *Headache*, **17**, 173–180.

46. Congdon, P.J. and Forsythe, W.I., (1979) Migraine in childhood: a study of 300 children. *Developmental Medicine and Child Neurology*, **21**, 209–216.

47. Jay, G.W. and Tomasi, L.G. (1981) Pediatric headaches: a one year retrospective analysis. *Headache*, **21**, 5–9.

48. Kurtz, A., Dilling, D., Blau, J.N. and Peckman, C. (1984) Migraine in children: findings from the national child development study, in *Progress in Migraine Research*, **2** (ed. F.C. Rose), Pittman Books, London, pp. 9–17.

2

Evaluation and classification

Andrew D. Hershey

When a patient first presents with a complaint of headache, the evaluation must start with a determination of the underlying etiology and subsequent diagnosis. This should include: a detailed history of the headaches, as well as the impact of other medical and social conditions; a detailed physical, neurological and comprehensive headache examination; and if any warning signs are present, further diagnostic testing may be indicated (Chapter 3). A practice parameter has been developed to address the evaluation of a child with headaches [1], with the history and examination being the most significant components of the evaluation. One of the first components of this evaluation is to identify if the headaches can be attributed to a secondary disorder (Chapters 14–17). If a secondary disorder is identified or suspected, then the treatment of this underlying factor should result in headache resolution. Headache classification schemes can be utilized to differentiate between primary and secondary headaches to assist with this identification. If treatment of this secondary disorder does not result in headache resolution, then the patient should be re-evaluated to see if the treatment was ineffective or if the patient had two separate disorders – the secondary disorder and a primary headache disorder. Only with proper evaluation and diagnostic identification can successful headache treatment outcomes be achieved.

2.1 Evaluation

The first step in the evaluation is the recognition of a problem with headaches in the first place. With the common nature and high prevalence of headaches, they

Pediatric Headaches in Clinical Practice   Andrew D. Hershey, Paul Winner, Marielle A. Kabbouche and Scott W. Powers
© 2009 John Wiley & Sons, Ltd.

are often underrecognized by patients, parents and health care providers. Secondary headaches may have a clear event that identifies the headache association (i.e. head trauma), but this may not be evident when the headache is recurrent. When the headaches are recurrent, patients and parents will often state 'Doesn't everybody get headache?' and will ignore or self-treat the problem. The headaches will then only become a recognized problem when these self-treatments are ineffective or the disability due to the headaches becomes a significant problem. Therefore, asking about headaches and pursuing the problem can assist the family and patient to identify the impact of the headaches and can result in improved diagnosis and disease recognition with subsequent improvement in treatment and overall outcome before it becomes a severe problem.

Once the presence of headache has been identified, a detailed headache history should be initiated. The headache history needs to be directed to both the patient and the parents. As pain symptomatology is individual and often subject to interpretation, a bias can exist by the examiner and the parent. It is essential, therefore, that the patient, a child, be completely involved in the history-taking process. Children can provide this useful information and essential information, but require that the questions are phrased at a developmentally appropriate level. When adolescents are involved, a separate interview may be needed. Use of questionnaires and a structured interview format that is developmentally appropriate can assist with this evaluation. If questionnaires are used to assist with the history taking, the responses need to be confirmed with the patient. As the parents often complete the questionnaire, they may interpret some of the answers based on their own experiences and observations that may vary from the patient's own experience.

The initial assessment is focused on whether this is a recurrent problem and, therefore, may be an episodic disorder and whether a secondary disorder is the cause. Oftentimes, a secondary headache disorder is clear from the inciting event, while at other times the parent or patient may assume a secondary cause when there is little direct evidence of this cause and effect. One clear example of this is with a diagnosis of sinus headache (Chapter 14). In this case, a primary headache disorder is often mistakenly diagnosed as a sinus headache and may have partial response to sinus treatment. The International Classification of Headache Disorders, 2nd edition (ICHD-II) [2] takes this into account by requiring that secondary headaches be directly attributed to the underlying etiology.

The detailed history can help identify the difference between primary and secondary headaches. Asking the patient to describe how long they have noticed having any headaches can begin to identify this difference. If the patient has had a long-standing history of recurrent headaches that have not changed in type, then the likelihood of a primary, recurrent headache disorder is increased. On the other hand, a new onset of headache or the development of a new headache type in a patient with recurrent headache raises the possibility of secondary headaches. Thus, duration of illness and a change in headache type can assist with the classification of the headache type.

The headache history needs to include a detailed description of the headache, including any premonitory symptoms, triggers or patterns. The presence of an aura needs to be addressed and may be an unusual concept for young children to understand. This is oftentimes complicated by migraine variants that need to be investigated (Chapter 9). Specific headache characteristics to address include cranial location of the pain (focal or diffuse), severity and quality of the pain, associated symptoms, frequency and duration of attacks, changes in or impact on activity level, and impact of the disease in terms of disability and quality of life.

For adults, the pain of a migraine may be identified as unilateral; however, in children it may be more likely to be bilateral, and a focal location may be more notable with a bifrontal or bitemple location being common [3]. A focal location is more consistent with migraine, whereas a diffuse location is associated with a tension-type headache.

A variety of tools can be utilized for severity assessment. This can include a categorical scale (e.g. mild, moderate or severe) or a numerical scale (e.g. 0–10). These appear to be equivalent for the assessment of severity for children with headaches [3], and choosing the most appropriate scale can be based on the developmental level of the child.

Associated symptoms have classically focused on the presence of nausea, vomiting, photophobia and phonophobia. Additional associated symptoms may also occur, including those related to autonomic changes seen in trigeminal autonomic cephalalgias (Chapter 12), specific brain locations, such as basilar-type migraine (Chapter 9), and the presence of cutaneous allodynia.

The frequency needs not only to address the number of headaches, but also the number of days per month, as long-duration headaches can affect multiple days. This can alter treatment choices. A headache that occurs on multiple days of the month but of long duration may need to focus on acute therapy, whereas frequent headaches of short duration may require a limit on the acute therapy and the initiation of preventative therapy. This can be further assessed with a characterization of the impact of the headaches on disability and the child's and family's quality of life (Chapter 5). Disability and headache impact can be assessed using standardized tools that are widely available [4–6].

The headache history also needs to include a detailed review of systems and past medical history, as well as a psychosocial and family history, in order to identify warnings. The medical history in the pediatric population should include details concerning pregnancy, labor and delivery, growth and development, previous injuries (especially head injuries), operations, hospitalizations, serious illnesses, drug allergies, current medications, and use of illicit drugs or alcohol. The past medical history can identify potential secondary causes, as well as potential co-morbid conditions that may affect response to treatment. Psychosocial stressors and school performance may also have an influence on the headache's impact and may provide a self-feedback mechanism for headache worsening. A family history of headaches is common for many of the primary headache disorders, although, as noted above, this may be discounted as a problem or the incorrect etiology may have been made by family members. It may, therefore, require a headache history of the family members present to achieve an accurate representation of the family history of headaches and their appropriate diagnosis.

Once the history has established the presence of a headache disorder, a complete physical, neurological and headache examination must be preformed. A practice parameter reviewed the evaluation of a child with headache and found that the most sensitive indicator of a need for further assessment is the neurological examination [1]. This should include a focus with special attention to gait abnormalities, since posterior fossa lesions will cause a wide-based, unsteady gait. The head circumference should be measured in young children. If significantly enlarged, then familial macrocephaly, hydrocephalus and neurofibromatosis are possibilities. The presence of a cranial bruit may indicate an underlying vascular abnormality. In young children, the fundu-scopic examination is best performed at the end of the examination with the room lights on to minimize the affect of a bright light and patient withdrawal, especially if the patient is photophobic.

If abnormalities on the neurological examination cannot be explained by medical history, then further investigation into the headache etiology is warranted, and neuroimaging is the most sensitive tool to detect a medically or surgically treatable cause.

A comprehensive headache exam may further help identify contributors to the headache's etiology [7]. This comprehensive headache exam can assist in identifying potential secondary causes, as well as be used to discuss with the family possible misconceptions as to the etiology of the headache. In the majority of patients with primary headaches, the general physical and neurologic examinations are normal, whereas there may be an abnormality on the examination with secondary headaches.

After completing a detailed history and medical examination, the practitioner should be able to determine whether the headaches are primary headaches or secondary headaches. Once secondary causes have been ruled out, the treatment of primary headaches can begin. If secondary headaches are suspected, then it is essential to treat the secondary cause. If the headaches persist after resolution of the secondary cause, then a reanalysis as to the etiology of the headaches must be considered.

In childhood, the most significant primary headache disorders brought to medical attention are migraine. This most commonly includes migraine without aura, probable migraine, migraine with aura, and chronic migraine.

2.2 Classification

With a complete headache history and through general, neurological and comprehensive headache examination, the key components to make an accurate diagnosis should be available. One key tool to help in this diagnosis is availability of established criteria. Standardized criteria have been developed with a variety of proposed classification schemes. Initially, these were anecdotally based on expert opinion. One of the most detailed criteria was established by the classification committee of the International Headache Society [8]. This classification was developed with the goal of describing all headache types and to be used for scientific and clinical diagnosis of headache disorders. It was initially based on a combination of historical descriptions and expert opinion, but with an intention that it be tested and revised over time. In this regard, the second edition was released in 2004 [2], with additional refinement anticipated over time.

ICHD-II divides headache into primary headaches, secondary headaches and cranial neuralgias. Primary headaches are those that are directly attributed to a neurological basis and include migraine, tension-type headaches and trigeminal autonomic cephalalgias (Table 2.1). Secondary headaches should be directly attributed to another medical condition. ICHD-II requires

Table 2.1 Primary headache disorders (ICHD-II criteria reproduced with permission from Blackwell Publishing)

Migraine (ICHD-II, 1)
    Migraine without aura (ICHD-II, 1.1)
    Migraine with aura (ICHD-II, 1.2)
    Childhood periodic syndromes (ICHD-II, 1.3)
    Retinal migraine (ICHD-II, 1.4)
    Complications of migraine (ICHD-II, 1.5)
    Chronic migraine (ICHD-II, 1.5.1)
    Status migrainosus (ICHD-II, 1.5.2)
    Probable migraine (ICHD-II, 1.6)

Tension-type headaches (ICHD-II, 2)
    Infrequent episodic tension-type headaches (ICHD-II, 2.1)
    Frequent episodic tension type headaches (ICHD-II, 2.2)
    Chronic tension-type headaches (ICHD-II, 2.3)
    Probable tension-type headaches (ICHD-II, 2.4)

Cluster headache and other trigeminal autonomic cephalalgias (ICHD-II, 3)
Other primary headaches (ICHD-II, 4)

a direct cause-and-effect relationship with the headaches resolving with treatment of the underlying secondary causes (Table 2.2). This is a change from the initial ICHD criteria, which only required an association. This association was often left up to interpretation and led to misdiagnoses.

Table 2.2 Secondary headache disorders[a] (ICHD-II criteria reproduced with permission from Blackwell Publishing)

Headaches attributed to head and/or neck trauma (ICHD-II, 5)
    Acute post-traumatic headaches (ICHD-II, 5.1)
    Chronic post-traumatic headaches (ICHD-II, 5.2)

Headaches attributed to cranial or cervical vascular disorders (ICHD-II, 6)
Headaches attributed to nonvascular intracranial disorders (ICHC-II, 7)
    Headaches attributed to high cerebrospinal fluid pressure (ICHD-II, 7.1)
    Headaches attributed to low cerebrospinal fluid pressure (ICHD-II, 7.2)
    Headaches attributed to intracranial neoplasm (ICHD-II, 7.4)
    Headaches attributed to epileptic seizure (ICHD-II, 7.6)
    Headaches attributed to Chiari malformation type I (ICHD-II, 7.7)

Headaches attributed to a substance or its withdrawal (ICHD-II, 8)
    Headaches induced by acute substance use or exposure (ICHD-II, 8.1)
    Medication-overuse headaches (ICHD-II, 8.2)
    Headache attributed to substance withdrawal (ICHD-II, 8.4)

Table 2.2 (*Continued*)

Headaches attributed to infection (ICHD-II, 9)
    Headaches attributed to intracranial infection (ICHD-II, 9.1)
    Headaches attributed to systemic infection (ICHD-II, 9.2)

Headaches attributed to disorders of homoeostasis (ICHD-II, 10)

Headaches or facial pain attributed to disorders of cranium, neck, eyes, ears, nose, sinuses, teeth, mouth or other facial or cranial structures (ICHD-II, 11)
    Headaches attributed to disorder of the eye (ICHD-II, 11.3)
    Headaches attributed to rhinosinusitis (ICHD-II, 11.5)

Headaches attributed to psychiatric disorders (ICHD-II, 12)

---

[a] Selected diagnoses.

The initial ICHD criteria were initially criticized for a lack of sensitivity and specificity in diagnosing childhood headaches, especially migraine. They were modified with footnotes to the criteria for migraine in ICHD-II [2]. This has improved the sensitivity, yet remains incomplete [3].

Some of the recognized problems for childhood migraine include the short duration, the bilateral location, the difficulty in describing the headache features and the evolution over time and developmental age [9]. Researchers have begun to examine additional tools for children to augment these criteria and include the use of drawings for young children [10, 11]. Regardless of these limitations, ICHD-II is the current foundation for the diagnosis and scientific study of headache and migraine.

References

1. Lewis, D.W., Ashwal, S., Dahl, G. *et al.* (2002) Practice parameter: evaluation of children and adolescents with recurrent headaches: report of the Quality Standards Subcommittee of the American Academy of Neurology and the Practice Committee of the Child Neurology Society. *Neurology*, **59**(4), 490–498.
2. Headache Classification Subcommittee of the International Headache Society (2004) The International Classification of Headache Disorders. *Cephalalgia: An International Journal of Headache*, **24**(Suppl. 1), 1–160.
3. Hershey, A.D., Winner, P., Kabbouche, M.A. *et al.* (2005) Use of the ICHD-II criteria in the diagnosis of pediatric migraine. *Headache*, **45**(10), 1288–1297.
4. Hershey, A.D., Powers, S.W., Vockell, A.L. *et al.* (2001) PedMIDAS: development of a questionnaire to assess disability of migraines in children. *Neurology*, **57**(11), 2034–2039.

5. Varni, J.W., Seid, M. and Kurtin, P.S. (2001) PedsQL 4.0: reliability and validity of the Pediatric Quality of Life Inventory version 4.0 generic core scales in healthy and patient populations. *Medical Care*, **39**(8), 800–812.

6. Powers, S.W., Patton, S.R., Hommel, K.A. and Hershey, A.D. (2003) Quality of life in childhood migraines: clinical impact and comparison to other chronic illnesses. *Pediatrics*, **112**(1 Pt 1), e1–e5.

7. Linder, S.L. (2005) Understanding the comprehensive pediatric headache examination. *Pediatric Annals*, **34**(6), 442–446.

8. Headache Classification Committee of the International Headache Society (1988) Classification and diagnostic criteria for headache disorders, cranial neuralgias and facial pain. *Cephalalgia: An International Journal of Headache*, **8**(S7), 1–96.

9. Virtanen, R., Aromaa, M., Rautava, P. *et al.* (2007) Changing headache from preschool age to puberty. A controlled study. *Cephalalgia: An International Journal of Headache*, **27**(4), 294–303.

10. Stafstrom, C.E., Goldenholz, S.R. and Dulli, D.A. (2005) Serial headache drawings by children with migraine: correlation with clinical headache status. *Journal of Child Neurology*, **20**(10), 809–813.

11. Stafstrom, C.E., Rostasy, K. and Minster, A. (2002) The usefulness of children's drawings in the diagnosis of headache. *Pediatrics*, **109**(3), 460–472.

3

Diagnostic testing and concerning variants

Marielle A. Kabbouche

The diagnosis of primary headache is a clinical diagnosis [1]. It is based on getting a detailed history and performing a thorough general and neurological examination.

Testing becomes necessary when a secondary-type headache is sus-pected, especially when the history, presentation or examinations are atypical [2].

This chapter will review most of the available tests and detail the need for appropriate requests. Reasons to order any test differ from practitioner to another. Guidelines are available and have been published by the American Academy of Neurology for adults and children after a thorough review of the literature [3–7].

Guidelines, as the term suggests, are necessary to *guide* our decisions in a clinical setting. A physician's role is to use the knowledge and experience they have acquired to individualize the care to each patient and specific clinical picture.

There is a lack of consensus concerning the role of diagnostic testing, including routine laboratory testing, lumbar puncture, electroencephalogram (EEG) and neuroimaging.

Pediatric Headaches in Clinical Practice   Andrew D. Hershey, Paul Winner, Marielle A. Kabbouche and Scott W. Powers
© 2009 John Wiley & Sons, Ltd.

The evaluation of a child with recurrent headache should include the following.

1. A detailed medical history:

   - date of birth;

   - age of onset of the symptoms;

   - description of the headache – including onset, type of pain, duration, triggers, associated symptoms, frequency;

   - medications used for the headache – acute therapy and the frequency per week where these medications are used, preventive medications taken and for how long, disability from headache;

   - past medical history and family history.

2. A thorough general examination, including vital signs and a full neurological and headache examination.

By the end of the evaluation the provider should be able, in most cases, to classify the headache into primary or secondary, as well as diagnose the subtype of the primary headache (migraine, chronic migraine, tension type headache, etc.).

The history of the headache may sometime be tricky to evaluate in young children. They frequently cannot describe the throbbing sensation, the photophobia, phonophobia or the occurrence of any 'migraine variant', which is a frequent complaint at this age but still an atypical presentation. These road blocks in the diagnosis of primary headache in young children explain the low threshold that clinicians have in ordering multiple testing.

One very effective and easy way to increase the chance in a clinical setting of getting a better history from a child is to give them a piece of paper to draw their headache. A study by Stafstrom *et al.* [8] in 2002 reviewed the sensitivity of picture drawing in the history taking in young children; 226 children drew a picture of their headache. The diagnosis was made by two pediatric neurologists. The first neurologist only used the pictures on which to base their diagnosis; the second neurologist made a clinical diagnosis.

The results of the study were very interesting and showed that the headache drawing by young children is 93.1% sensitive in the diagnosis of headache and 82.7% specific.

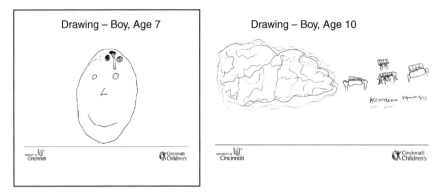

Figure 3.1 Pounding Headache.

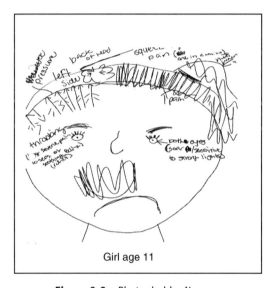

Figure 3.2 Photophobia, Nausea.

The drawings were very descriptive of the symptoms occurring during the headache, even when the patient refrained from describing them clinically. This included the pounding sensation, visual phenomena, gastroenterological symptoms and focal neurological symptoms (Figures 3.1 and 3.2).

At the end of the clinical evaluation, the clinician should be confident of making a decision on the final diagnosis or the necessity of further testing.

The diagnostic testing available for headache includes the following, which are discussed below:

- neuroimaging;

- electroencephalogram;

- lumbar puncture;

- clinical laboratory testing.

3.1 Neuroimaging

The reasons for considering any type of neuroimaging for headache were reviewed and published by Evans [9] and included the following guidelines.

Imaging is necessary if one of the following is present during the clinical interview:

- subacute headache with rapidly progressive increase in severity;

- new onset headache in immunosuppressed patient;

- headache of new onset in patient older then 50 years old;

- first or worst headache;

- associated systemic symptoms, such as fever, nuchal rigidity, etc.;

- headache with focal neurological abnormalities on physical examination.

These guidelines cover the general population. Other factors should be considered in the decision to image in children due to specific headache types, presentations and pathologies at this age.

Medina *et al.* [10] reviewed imaging and testing in children. The results of their study revealed that the highest leads in brain imaging were found in a specific high-risk group. This group can be separated from others clinically.

Children in this group had at least one of the following for 'space-occupying lesion' predictive values:

- headache of less than 1 month duration;

- absence of family history of migraine/primary headache;

- abnormal neurological examination;

- gait abnormalities;

- seizures;

- sleep-related headaches, vomiting and confusion.

The American Academy of Neurology published its practice parameters on neuroimaging use in the evaluation of headache in adults in 1994 for when a neurological examination is normal. This was based on 897 adults in multiple studies through a thorough literature review of computed tomography (CT) scanning and magnetic resonance imaging (MRI) scans. The American Academy of Neurology statement was that imaging is not warranted in patients with *recurrent* migraine headaches with *no* change in pattern, *no* history of seizure and *no* other focal neurological signs [5–7].

How about recommendations for headache in children?

A literature search and review of neuroimaging in children similar to that for adults was done [7]. The studies included altogether 116 CT scans, 483 MRI scans and 75 using both techniques.

Imaging abnormalities found were as follows:

- 16% had incidental, nonsurgical findings, including Chiari malformation, arachnoid cysts without mass effect, pranasal sinus disease, occult vascular abnormalities, others (cavum septi, pineal cyst, ventricular asymmetry, etc.);

- 3% of children had a surgically treatable lesion or lesion necessitating medical intervention, such as a pituitary gland abnormality;

- only 10 patients had a tumor, including medulloblastoma, cerebrellar astrocytoma, choroind plexus papilloma, sarcoma, primitive neuroectodermal tumor (PNET), glioblastoma.

The risk of having a space-occupying lesion was similar to what is described earlier as predictive values by Medina *et al.* [10], including a headache of less than 1 month duration, no family history of primary headaches, an abnormal neurological examination, gait abnormalities, seizures, sleep-related headaches, vomiting and confusion.

The recommendations for children were reported by the quality standards subcommittee of the American Academy of Neurology and the Practice Committee of the Child Neurology Society [7]. The guidelines were as follows:

Table 3.1   Summary of general guidelines for requesting imaging in children with headache

1   Abnormal neurological examination
2   Atypical presentation of the headache: vertigo, intractable vomiting, headache waking the child from sleep
3   Recent headache of less than 6 months
4   Child of less then 6 years of age
5   No family history of migraine and or primary headache
6   Occipital headache
7   Change in type of headache
8   Subacute progressive headache severity
9   New onset headache in an immunosuppressed child
10 First and/or worst headache
11 Systemic symptoms and signs
12 Headache associated with confusion, mental status changes or focal neurological complaints

- Obtaining a neuroimaging on a routine basis is not indicated in children with recurrent headache and a normal neurological examination.

- Neuroimaging should be considered in children with an abnormal neurological examination and in whom there are historical features suggesting recent onset of headache, change in the type of headache, neurological dysfunction, occipital location of the headache.

Table 3.1 summarizes the general guidelines for requesting imaging in children with headache.

What imaging technique should one use when requesting neuroimaging: CT or MRI? A CT scan is a fast imaging technique that is widely used in emergency rooms. It is highly sensitive in acute hemorrhage. However, an MRI scan is more sensitive in evaluating the posterior fossa, an area of high incidence of pathology in children. An MRI scan of the brain is also more sensitive to neoplastic disorders, vascular disorders, ischemia and infection.

The recommendation would be to request an MRI scan if an imaging is considered necessary unless an acute hemorrhage is suspected.

3.2 EEG

An EEG was previously frequently used in the diagnosis of headache [11–13]. The only significant abnormality reported in primary headache patients was a prominent response during photic stimulation called the 'H' response [14]. This driving response did not differentiate between all types of primary headache and was present in migraine-type and tension-type headaches, and so the use of the EEG in adults was considered of no value for the diagnosis of migraine.

There are no studies available that clearly compare the incidence of EEG abnormalities in migraine versus a nonmigraine headache in the pediatric population.

What is interesting in children, especially young ones, is the richness of atypical symptoms, including periodic symptoms and migraine variants. These migraine precursors can occur without an apparent headache and can clinically present as a seizure disorder.

In these cases an EEG is warranted not for the diagnosis of headache, but to evaluate for a possible underlying seizure disorder.

Hence, to summarize:

1. An EEG is not recommended in the routine evaluation of a child with recurrent headache, as it is unlikely to provide an etiology or improve the diagnostic yield in primary headache.

2. An EEG would be of value to evaluate for any suspected seizure, epilepsy or postictal headache [3].

3.3 Lumbar puncture

A lumbar puncture is usually necessary in the following clinical presentations:

– infection;

– suspected increased intracranial pressure (papilledema);

– suspicion of a subarachnoid hemorrhage with normal CT head.

If a lumbar puncture is requested, then it is imperative *always* to measure an opening pressure. This issue is delicate, especially in children, since a false positive of a high measurement can occur if the child is not relaxed with hands and legs extended.

Indications for a lumbar puncture in the evaluation of headache in children include [4]:

1. first and/or worst headache to rule out a subarachnoid hemorrhage, especially if suspicion is high and the CT scanning is negative;

2. headache with fever/nuchal rigidity or other signs of meningismus;

3. headache in an immunosuppressed patient;

4. evaluation for increased/decreased intracranial pressure (pseudotumor cerebri/low-pressure headache).

Otherwise, a lumbar puncture is not indicated for routine diagnosis of a primary headache, including migraine

3.4 Clinical laboratory testing

Clinical laboratory studies are not needed in the routine evaluation of primary headache.

When requested, these tests usually target a baseline cell count to rule out an underlying anemia that can be at the origin of headaches and thyroid hormones if hypo/hyperthyroidism is suspected.

Routine baseline testing can also be of value prior to initiating preventive headache medications, as well as in monitoring their toxicity and compliance on these drugs [15].

References

1. Bille, B. (1962) Migraine in school children. *Acta Paediatrica (Oslo, Norway: 1992)*, **51**(Suppl 136), 1–151.
2. Lewis, D.W. (2001) Headache in the pediatric emergency department, in *Headaches in Children and Adolescents* (eds P. Winner and A.D. Rothner), B.C. Decker, Inc., Hamilton, pp. 163–181.
3. Quality Standards Subcommittee of the American Academy of Neurology (1995) Practice parameter: the electroencephalogram in the evaluation of headache (summary statement). Report of the Quality Standards Subcommittee of the American Academy of Neurology. *Neurology* **45**, 1411–1413.
4. Quality Standards Subcommittee of the American Academy of Neurology (1993) Practice parameters: lumbar puncture (summary statement). Report of the Quality Standards Subcommittee of the American Academy of Neurology. *Neurology*, **43**, 625–627.

5. Quality Standards Subcommittee of the American Academy of Neurology (1994) Practice parameter: the utility of neuroimaging in the evaluation of headache in patients with normal neurologic examinations (summary statement). Report of the Quality Standards Subcommittee of the American Academy of Neurology. *Neurology*, **44**, 1353–1354.

6. Silberstein, S.D. (2000) Practice parameter: evidence-based guidelines for migraine headache (an evidence-based review): report of the Quality Standards Subcommittee of the American Academy of Neurology. *Neurology*, **55**, 754–762.

7. Lewis, D.W., Ashwal, S., Dahl, G. *et al.* (2002) Practice parameter: evaluation of children and adolescents with recurrent headaches: report of the Quality Standards Subcommittee of the American Academy of Neurology and the Practice Committee of the Child Neurology Society. *Neurology*, **59**(4), 490–498.

8. Stasftrom, C.E., Rostary, K. and Minster, A. (2002) Usefulness of children's drawings in the diagnosis of headache. *Pediatrics*, **109**(3), 460–472.

9. Evans, R. (2001) Diagnostic testing for headache. *Medical Clinics of North America*, **85**(4), 865–885.

10. Medina, L.S., D'Souza, B. and Vasconcellos, E. (2003) Adults and children with headache: evidence-based diagnostic evaluation. *Neuroimaging Clinics of North America*, **13**(2), 225–235.

11. Chen, J.H., Wang, P.J., Young, C. *et al.* (1994) Etiological classification of chronic headache in children and their electroencephalographic features. *Acta Paediatrica Scandinavica*, **35**, 397–406.

12. Kramer, U., Nevo, Y. and Harel, S. (1997) Electroencephalography in the evaluation of headache patients: a review. *Israel Journal of Medical Sciences*, **33**, 816–820.

13. Kramer, U., Nevo, Y., Neufeld, M.Y. *et al.* (1994) The value of EEG in children with chronic headaches. *Brain & Development*, **16**, 304–308.

14. Whitehouse, D., Pappas, J.A., Escala, P.H. et al. (1967) Electroencephalographic changes in children with migraine. *The New England Journal of Medicine*, **276**, 23–27.

15. Sargent, J.D. and Solbach, P. (1983) Medical evaluation of migraineurs: review of the value of laboratory and radiologic tests. *Headache*, **23**, 62–65.

4
Epidemiology of pediatric headache

Paul Winner

Pediatric headache disorders carry a high incidence and prevalence along with an economic burden both to the patient and their parents. An accurate system for their diagnosis and classification is an important priority for both clinical practice and research [1]. Various classification schemes have been proposed for headache disorders in adolescents and children. The criteria proposed by the International Headache Society represent a significant advance, although these criteria were developed primarily for headache disorders in adults [2, 3]. The emerging criteria provide important tools for epidemiologic research [4–9]. In the absence of an accepted diagnostic standard, clinicians and researchers have struggled to develop valid and reliable diagnostic criteria for this population [10]. The lack of standardized case definitions has plagued epidemiologic studies of pediatric headache and has contributed to the enormous variation in estimates of the prevalence and incidence of pediatric headache disorders [11–13]. Headaches undergo exacerbations, transformations and remissions in childhood.

Epidemiologists must rely on the recall of patients or parents; thus, diagnoses are subject to recall bias [14–18]. This chapter will focus on the epidemiology of migraine in the pediatric population, since we have the most data for this population.

Pediatric Headaches in Clinical Practice   Andrew D. Hershey, Paul Winner, Marielle A. Kabbouche and Scott W. Powers
© 2009 John Wiley & Sons, Ltd.

4.1 Epidemiology of migraine

We know that migraine is one of the most burdensome of the primary headache disorders in the pediatric population. Epidemiologic data help to describe the burden of migraine as well as its scope and distribution. Understanding sociodemographic, genetic and environmental risk factors helps identify those groups at highest risk for migraine and may provide clues to the disease mechanisms, classification and/or treatment.

4.2 Incidence

Incidence refers to the rate of onset of the new cases of a particular disease in a defined population. The incidence of migraine is best evaluated in longitudinal studies [19]. Stewart *et al.* [20] estimated the migraine incidence using the reported age of onset from a prevalence study. In males, the incidence of migraine with aura peaked around 5 years of age at 6.6/1000 person-years; the peak for migraine without aura was 10/1000 person-years between 10 and 11 years. New cases of migraine were uncommon in men in their 30s. In females, the incidence of migraine with aura peaked between ages 12 and 13 years (14.1/ 1000 person-years); migraine without aura peaked between ages 14 and 17 years (18.9/1000 person-years). Thus, migraine seems to begin earlier in males than in females, and migraine with aura seems to begin earlier than migraine without aura [20].

In a study by Stang *et al.* [21], the overall age-adjusted incidence was 137 per 100 000 person-years for males and 294 per 100 000 person-years for females. The highest incidence in females was among those aged 20 to 24 years (689 per 100 000 person-years), and the highest incidence in males was among those aged 10 to 14 years (246 per 100 000 person-years). More recently, a large study by Stewart *et al.* [22] has suggested that the cumulative lifetime risk of migraine is substantially higher than estimates of 1-year prevalence and that the median age of onset occurs long after puberty for both males and females than previously reported, suggesting that migraine may begin later and be shorter than pre-viously thought.

4.3 Prevalence

The reported prevalence of migraine varied widely, probably because of differences in the methodology and classifications used [22–24]. Before pub-erty, migraine prevalence is higher in boys than in girls, although recent data [1, 25] from the American Migraine Prevalence and Prevention (AMPP) study challenge this paradigm; as adolescence approaches, the incidence and prevalence increase more rapidly in girls than in boys. The prevalence increases throughout childhood and early adult life until approximately age 40 years, after which it declines [20]. The female-to-male migraine prevalence ratio varies with age. The onset of hormonal changes associated with menses may contribute to this variation. Hormonal factors cannot be the sole cause; differences persist to age 70 years and later, well beyond the time that cyclical hormonal changes can be considered a factor [20, 26].

The relationship between migraine prevalence and socioeconomic status is uncertain. In clinic-based studies, migraine appears to be associated with high intelligence and social class. In Bille's [27, 28] studies of children, he did not find any association between migraine prevalence and intelligence. Similarly, in adults, epidemiologic studies do not support a relationship between occupation and migraine prevalence [24, 25, 29]. In both the American Migraine Study I and II, migraine prevalence was inversely related to household income. Migraine prevalence fell as household income increased [24, 25]. This inverse relationship between migraine and socioeconomic status was confirmed in another US study based on members of a managed care organization and in the National Health Interview Study, and recent data from the AMPP [25]. Migraine prevalence also varies by race and geography. In the USA, it is highest in Caucasians, intermediate in African Americans, and lowest in Asian Americans. Similarly, a meta-analysis of prevalence studies suggests that migraine is most common in North and South America, similar in Europe, but lower in Africa, and often lowest in studies from Asia [21]. The influence of reporting bias on these findings cannot be excluded. Nonetheless, the data suggest that race-related differences in genetic risk may contribute. Whether and how these differences apply to the pediatric population, or whether these differences have later expression, are still to be determined.

The prevalence of headache in children has been investigated in a number of school and population-based studies. By age 3 years, headache occurs in 3–8% of children. At age 5 years, 19.5% have headache; and by age 7 years, 37–51.5% have headaches. In 7- to 15-year-olds, headache prevalence ranges from 57 to 82% [17, 30–34]. The prevalence increases from ages 3 to 11 years in both boys and girls, with a higher headache prevalence in 3- to 5-year-old boys than in 3- to 5-year-old girls [7, 32–34]. The overall prevalence of headache increases from preschool-age children to mid-adolescence when examined using various cross-sectional studies [17, 30–34]. Raieli *et al.* [18] assessed the prevalence of migraine headache in an epidemiologic survey of 11- to 14-year-old students. The sample was selected from a population registry for an Italian city. Students were interviewed by neurologists at school using semistructured interviews. The authors found that headache prevalence was stable in boys, while it increased uniformly in girls. Overall migraine prevalence was 3.0%, with a slight female preponderance [18].

The study of Raieli *et al.* found a lower prevalence than other studies in this age group. A study performed in the UK showed that migraine prevalence was higher in boys than in girls at 3–5 years of age and at 5–7 years of age [7]. Prevalence was equal in boys and girls at 7 to 11 years and was higher in girls after age 11.7 years.

Two studies reported the prevalence of pediatric migraine in the Middle East. The first one, performed in southern Iran, evaluated a random sample of 1868 teenaged girls (aged 11–18 years) with 507 reported headaches. The overall prevalence rate for migraine was 6.1% (95% confidence interval (CI): 5.0–7.2) and for tension-type headache, 12.1% (95% CI: 10.6–13.6). Migraine and tension-type headaches were significantly associated. The exposition of subjects to sunlight, type of food and a family history of headache were the most significant factors associated with migraine and tension-type headaches [35]. The second study evaluated 1400 randomly selected Saudi children in grades 1 through 9. Overall, the headache prevalence was 49.8%. The prevalence of migraine was 7.1%. For both boys and girls, the age-specific prevalence rate for nonmigraine headache rose steadily from around 15% at age 6–7 years to nearly 60% after age 15 years. For migraine, there was a sharp increase in the prevalence rate (from around 2% to around 9%) at age 10–11 years, also in both boys and girls. Age-adjusted prevalence for migraine between age 6 and 15 years was 6.2% [36]. A study evaluated the evolution over 5 years of juvenile migraine without aura in adolescents. Sixty-four subjects out of 80 previously selected were reevaluated [37]. Thirty-two (50%) had migraine without aura. After 5 years, migraine without aura persisted in 56.2%, converted to a probable migraine or nonclassifiable headache in 9.4% and 3.1% of cases respectively, changed to episodic tension-type headache in 12.5%, and remitted in 18.8% [37].

4.4 The AMPP study

The AMPP study is the largest population study on migraine conducted to date. In the AMPP study, a total of 120 000 households, from a panel of households representative of the US population, were assessed. The AMPP study is a multiyear longitudinal study that, among several other headache-related aims, evaluates the epidemiology, the burden and the patterns of health care utilization for migraine [1]. As a part of the AMPP study, adolescents were also investigated, yielding data for 18 714 individuals aged 12–19 years. An overall 1-year period prevalence of 6.3% was reported. The prevalence in boys was 5.0%; in girls it was 7.7% [1]. The adjusted prevalence in boys was remarkably stable, ranging from 2.9 to 4.1%. It did not significantly differ in any age. In girls, compared with the age of 12 years, the prevalence was significantly higher in those at older ages. For both genders, the prevalence was significantly higher in Caucasians than in African Americans [1]. Population studies show that individuals from high-income groups were much more likely to report a medical diagnosis of migraine than those with lower income [1, 25]. It has been discussed that perhaps migraine is a disease of persons with high income in the doctor's office because high-income individuals seek care. As suggested, people from higher income households are more likely to consult physicians and, therefore, are disproportionately included in clinic-based studies [1, 25]. The higher prevalence in the lower socioeconomic groups may, alternatively, be a consequence of a circumstance associated with low income and migraine, such as poor diet, poor medical care or stress. It may also reflect social selection; that is, migraineurs may have lower incomes because migraine interferes with educational and occupational function, causing a loss of income or the ability to rise from a low-income group [1, 25]. In the AMPP study there was a strong, consistent inverse relationship between migraine prevalence in adolescents and household income just when the parents did not have migraine. The inverse relationship disappeared when the parents have migraine. It is postulated that, in the presence of biological predisposition, environmental risk factors were less evident. When biological predisposition was less evident, social causation explained the inverse relationship [1, 25].

4.5 Disability

A minority (25.6%) of adolescents with migraine had less than one severe headache day per month, while most (61%) had from one to four. Similar to what is seen in adults, most adolescents reported severe impairment (60.8%) during migraine attacks, while just 6.2% reported no impairment at all [1].

Over a 3-month period, 41.1% of the migraineurs had at least 1 day of limitation related to the headache. Although in the population, as expected, most adolescents (71.6%) were classified as having no or little migraine-related disability, a total of 16.3% had moderate or severe disability levels [1]. More interestingly, adolescents lost a mean of 6.95 days of reduced productivity over a 3-month period [1].

4.6 Treatment issues

Most adolescents surveyed by the AMPP study treated their attacks with over-the-counter (OTC) medicines only (59.3%), while 16.5% used prescription medication most of the time and 22.1% used both OTC medicines and prescription medication for their acute treatment. Using acute prescription medication was more common in females, Caucasians and individuals with increasing age [1].

The majority of them (63.7%) never used a migraine preventive treatment and just 10.6% were currently using it. Another 6.3% were using medications that are effective for migraine prevention for other reasons, and 19.5% had used medications in the past but were not currently using them [1].

4.7 Other primary headaches

Tension-type headaches are generally considered mild recurrent headaches, and many features are the opposite of migraine. Epidemiology studies have varied on the prevalence of these headaches in children due to the present criteria.

Cluster headaches can begin at any age; the mean age of onset is approximately late 20s. Childhood and adolescent onset cluster headaches have been reported, but these early onset cases appear to be rare. Only 18% of patients had their onset of cluster headaches prior to age 18 years and 2% began before the age of 10 years [38].

4.8 Conclusions

The process of diagnosis and classification in children, adolescents and adults is fundamentally similar, though there are differences in the details [39–43]. If secondary headache is not present, then the clinician proceeds to diagnose a specific primary headache disorder. It is important to recognize that migraine in children is often of short duration. Another important issue is in regard to the male predominance prior to puberty, which changes to a situation of female predominance after puberty. Children with migraine seem to have fewer attacks per month, with a higher number of daytime attacks than adults. Their attacks tend to be shorter, less severe and easier to treat. They are often relieved by sleep and are more easily controlled. As children enter adolescence, their migraines begin to resemble the adult phenotype. The onset of hormonal changes associated with menses may contribute to the female prevalence observed beyond adolescence. Specifically, estrogen withdrawal may trigger migraine [26]. The lack of standardized case definitions continues to plague epidemiologic studies of pediatric headache and contributes to the variation in estimates of the prevalence and incidence of pediatric headache disorders.

References

1. Bigal, M.E., Lipton, R.B., Winner, P., Reed, M.L., Diamond, S., and Stewart, W.F. (2007) Migraine in adolescents: association with socioeconomic status and family history. *Neurology*, **69**(1), 16–25.

2. International Headache Society (1988) Classification and diagnostic criteria for headache disorders, cranial neuralgias, and facial pain. *Cephalalgia: An International Journal of Headache*, **8** (Suppl 7), 1–96.

3. Hershey, A.D., Winner, P., Kabbouche, M.A. *et al.* (2005) Use of the ICHD-II criteria in the diagnosis of pediatric migraine. *Headache*, **45**(10), 1288–1297.

4. Gallai, V., Sarchielli, P., Carboni, F. *et al.* (1995) Applicability of the 1988 IHS criteria to headache patients under the age of 18 years attending 21 Italian headache clinics. *Headache*, **35**, 146–153.

5. Rothner, D.A. and Winner, P. (2001) Headaches in children and adolescents, in *Wolff's Headache and Other Head Pain*, 7th edn (eds S.D. Silberstein, R.B. Lipton and D.J. Dalessio), Oxford University Press, New York, pp. 539–561.

6. Maytal, J., Young, M., Schechter, A. and Lipton, R.B. (1997) Pediatric migraine and the International Headache Society (IHS) criteria. *Neurology*, **48**, 602–607.

7. Mortimer, J., Kay, J. and Jaron, A. (1992) Epidemiology of headache and childhood migraine in an urban general practice using ad hoc, Vahlquist and IHS criteria. *Developmental Medicine and Child Neurology*, **34**, 1095–1101.

8. Seshia, S., Wolstein, J., Adams, C. *et al.* (1994) International Headache Society criteria and childhood headache. *Developmental Medicine and Child Neurology*, **36**, 419–428.

9. Wober-Bingol, C., Wober, C., Karwautz, A. *et al.* (1995) Diagnosis of headache in children and adolescence: a study in 437 patients. *Cephalalgia: An International Journal of Headache*, **15**, 13–21.

10. Lipton, R.B. and Stewart, W.F. (1997) Prevalence and impact of migraine. *Neurologic Clinics*, **15**, 1–13.

11. Lipton, R.B., Stewart, W.F. and Merikangas, K. (1993) Reliability in headache diagnosis. *Cephalalgia: An International Journal of Headache*, **13** (Suppl 12), 29–33.

12. Merikangas, K.R., Angst, J. and Isler, H. (1990) Migraine and psychopathology: results of the Zurich cohort study of young adults. *Archives of General Psychiatry*, **47**, 849–853.

13. Merikangas, K.R. and Frances, A. (1993) Development of diagnostic criteria for headache syndromes: lessons from psychiatry. *Cephalalgia: An International Journal of Headache*, **13** (Suppl 12), 34–38.

14. Lint, M.S. and Steart, W.F. (1984) Migraine headache: epidemiologic perspectives. *Epidemiologic Reviews*, **6**, 107–139.

15. Gladstein, J., Holden, E.W., Perotta, L. and Raven, M. (1993) Diagnosis and symptom-patterns in children presenting to a pediatric headache clinic. *Headache*, **33**, 497–500.

16. Abu-Arefeh, I. and Russell, G. (1994) Prevalence of headache and migraine in school children. *BMJ (Clinical Research)*, **309**, 765–769.

17. Bille, B. (1962) Migraine in school children. *Acta Paediatrica Scandinavica*, **51** (Suppl 136), 1–151.

18. Raieli, V., Raimondo, D., Cammalleri, R. and Camarda, R. (1995) Migraine headache in adolescents: a student population-based study in Monreale. *Cephalalgia: An International Journal of Headache*, **15**, 5–12.

19. Cummings, R.G., Kelsy, J.L. and Nevitt, M.C. (1990) Methodologic issues in the study of frequent and recurrent health problems. *Annals of Epidemiology*, **1**, 49–56.

20. Stewart, W.F., Linet, M.S., Celentano, D.D. *et al.* (1993) Age and sex-specific incidence rates of migraine with and without visual aura. *American Journal of Epidemiology*, **34**, 1111–1120.

21. Stang, P.E., Yanagihara, T., Swanson, J.W. *et al.* (1992) Incidence of migraine headaches: a population-based study in Olmstead County, Minnesota. *Neurology*, **42**, 1657–1662.

22. Stewart, W.F., Simon, D., Schechter, A. and Lipton, R.B. (1995) Population variation in migraine prevalence: a meta-analysis. *Journal of Clinical Epidemiology*, **48**, 269–280.

23. Rasmussen, B.K. (1995) Epidemiology of headache. *Cephalalgia: An International Journal of Headache*, **15**, 45–68.

24. Lipton, R.B., Hamelsky, S.W. and Hamelsky, S.W. (2001) Epidemiology and impact of headache, in *Wolff's Headache and Other Head Pain*, 7th edn (eds S.D. Silberstein, R.B. Lipton and D.J. Dalessio), Oxford University Press, New York, pp. 85–107.

25. Diamond, S., Bigal, M.E., Silberstein, S., *et al.* (2007) Patterns of diagnosis and acute and preventive treatment of migraine in the United States. Results of the American Migraine Prevalence and Prevention Study. *Headache* **47**(9), 1365.

26. Silberstein, S.D. (1992) The role of sex hormones in headache. *Neurology*, **42** (Suppl 2), 37–42.

27. Bille, B. (1981) Migraine in childhood and its prognosis. *Cephalalgia: An International Journal of Headache*, **1**, 71–75.

28. Bille, B. (1989) Migraine in children: prevalence, clinical features, and a 30-year follow up, in *Migraine and Other Headaches* (eds M.D. Ferrari and X. Lataste), Parthenon, Park Ridge, NJ.

29. Lipton, R.B., Stewart, W.F. and Simon, D. (1998) Medical consultation for migraine: results from the American Migraine Study. *Headache*, **38**(2), 87–96.

30. Sillanpää, M. (1983) Changes in the prevalence of migraine and other headaches during the first seven school years. *Headache*, **23**, 15–19.

31. Sillanpää, M. and Antilla, P. (1996) Increasing prevalence of headache in 7-year-old school children. *Headache*, **36**, 466–470.

32. Sillanpää, M., Piekkala, P. and Kero, P. (1991) Prevalence of headache at preschool age in an unselected child population. *Cephalalgia: An International Journal of Headache*, **11**, 239–242.

33. Sillanpää, M. and Piekkala, P. (1984) Prevalence of migraine and other headaches in early puberty. *Scandinavian Journal of Primary Health Care*, **2**, 27–32.

34. Sillanpää, M. (1983) Prevalence of headache in prepuberty. *Headache*, **23**, 10–14.

35. Ayatollahi, S.M., Moradi, F. and Ayatollahi, S.A. (2002) Prevalences of migraine and tension-type headache in adolescent girls of Shiraz (southern Iran). *Headache*, **42**(4), 287–290.

36. Al Jumah, M., Awada, A. and Al Azzam, S. (2002) Headache syndromes amongst schoolchildren in Riyadh, Saudi Arabia. *Headache*, **42**(4), 281–286.

37. Guidetti, V. and Galli, F. (1998) Evolution of headache in childhood and adolescence: an 8-year follow-up. *Cephalalgia: An International Journal of Headache*, **18**, 449–454.

38. Newman, L.C. and Maytal, J. (2008) Epidemiology and impact of headache, in *Headache in Children and Adolescents*, 2nd edn (eds P. Winner, D.W. Lewis and A.D. Rothner), BC Decker, Hamilton, ON, pp. 147–161.

39. Ozge, A., Bugdayci, R., Sasmaz, T. *et al.* (2002) The sensitivity and specificity of the case definition criteria in diagnosis of headache: a school-based epidemiological study of 5562 children in Mersin. *Cephalalgia: An International Journal of Headache*, **22**(10), 791–798.

40. Ottman, R., Hong, S. and Lipton, R.B. (1993) Validity of family history data on severe headache and migraine. *Neurology*, **43**, 1954–1960.

41. Winner, P.K. (2001) The young girl with incapacitating headache, in *Advanced Therapy of Headache* (eds A.M. Rapoport, F.D. Sheftell and R.A. Purdy), BC Decker, Hamilton, ON, pp. 23–30.

42. Sillanpää, M. (1979) Prevalence of migraine and other headache in Finnish children starting school. *Headache*, **15**, 288–290.

43. Zuckerman, B., Stevenson, J. and Bailey, V. (1987) Stomachaches and headaches in a community sample of preschool children. *Pediatrics*, **79**, 677–682.

5
Impact of childhood headaches

Scott W. Powers

This chapter will briefly summarize what is known about the impact of childhood headache in terms of quality of life, disability and psychosocial functioning. Also, suggestions for how to incorporate evidence-based assessments of headache impact into clinical practice will be provided.

5.1 Childhood headache and quality of life

It is clear that, for children with headaches, quality of life is impacted. Indeed, many children with headache report that their pain is debilitating. For example, in children with migraine who seek treatment, the negative impact on quality of life of their headache is similar to that of children with arthritis and cancer, with the most profound impairments in school and emotional functioning [1]. While the majority of children with headache do not experience significant changes in psychosocial functioning, there appears to be a subset of children for whom headache pain not only causes immediate impact, but also has more broad psychosocial effects, increasing risk for academic difficulties, and emotional problems such as depression and anxiety [2]. In addition, a notable subset of children with headache continues to experience significant headaches into adulthood [3–5]. When a child or adolescent presents with headache, it is imperative to consider how this pain is impacting the individual and their family and to assume, based upon current data, that the impact is clinically significant.

Pediatric Headaches in Clinical Practice   Andrew D. Hershey, Paul Winner, Marielle A. Kabbouche and Scott W. Powers
© 2009 John Wiley & Sons, Ltd.

5.2 Evidence-based assessment in clinical practice

In clinical practice, management of children and adolescents with headache should incorporate the addition of headache disability and quality of life assessments to the traditional outcomes of headache intensity, duration and frequency. We add a headache disability measure specifically designed for use in pediatrics, the PedMIDAS [6], and a general quality of life measure that is applicable for children aged 2 to 18 years, the Pediatric Quality of Life Inventory Version 4.0 (PedsQL) [1]. The reliability, validity and utility of these measures have been demonstrated, and they can be efficiently incorporated into day-to-day clinical care [7–9]. The measures are complementary, showing a correlation of 0.34, and both add unique information to the determination of the outcome of intervention. Assessments should occur at initial evaluation and regularly throughout treatment. Results are communicated with the children and their families, as well as described in correspondence with other health care providers, such as the child's pediatrician. Notably, we discuss with children and adolescents that our ultimate goal for their headache care is to achieve a level of disability in the little to none category [7] and a level of quality of life that is comparable to normative values for healthy children [1].

5.3 Summary

The experience of headache by children impacts their lives. This impact can be measured and the data that are obtained should be used in the clinical care of these patients. It is important to assess disability and quality of life as components of an evidence-based approach to clinical care of these children and their families.

References

1. Powers, S.W., Patton, S.R., Hommel, K.A. and Hershey, A.D. (2003) Quality of life in childhood migraines: clinical impact and comparison to other chronic illnesses. *Pediatrics*, **112**, e1–e5. Accessed on 13 January 2004 at http://www.pediatrics.org/cgi/content/full/112/1/e1.

2. Powers, S.W., Kruglak-Gilman, D. and Hershey, A.D. (2006) Headache and psychosocial functioning in children and adolescents. *Headache*, **46**, 1404–1415.

3. Andrasik, F. and Schwartz, M.S. (2006) Behavioral assessment and treatment of pediatric headache. *Behavior Modification*, **30**(1), 93–113.

4. Brna, P., Dooley, J., Gordon, K. and Dewan, T. (2005) The prognosis of childhood headache: a 20-year follow-up. *Archives of Pediatrics & Adolescent Medicine*, **159**, 1157–1160.

5. Connelly, M. (2003) Recurrent pediatric headache: a comprehensive review. *Child Health Care*, **32**(3), 153–189.

6. Hershey, A.D., Powers, S.W., Vockell, A.-L. *et al.* (2001) PedMIDAS: development of a questionnaire to assess disability of migraines in children. *Neurology*, **57**, 2034–2039.

7. Hershey, A.D., Powers, S.W., Vockell, A.-L. *et al.* (2004) Development of a patient-based grading scale for PedMIDAS. *Cephalalgia: An International Journal of Headache*, **24**, 844–849.

8. Powers, S.W., Patton, S.R., Hommel, K.A. and Hershey, A.D. (2004) Quality of life in pediatric migraine: characterization of age-related effects using PedsQL 4.0. *Cephalalgia: An International Journal of Headache*, **24**, 120–127.

9. Powers, S.W., Kruglak-Gilman, D., Hershey, A.D. and The Headache Center Team at Cincinnati Children's Hospital (2006) Clinical Pearl/Brief Report: suggestions for a biopsychosocial approach to treating children and adolescents who present with headache. *Headache*, **46**(Suppl 3), S149–S150.

6

Emergent evaluation and management

Marielle A. Kabbouche

Headache is one of the most common presenting complaints to emergency departments (EDs). It is the third leading cause of referral to a pediatric emergency room [1]. The overwhelming majority of headaches are benign in nature and can be accurately diagnosed on the basis of a careful history and physical examination. Headache can, however, be the initial symptom of life-threatening disorders presenting to an emergency room, such as meningitis, intracranial hemorrhage, brain tumor or hydrocephalus.

It is essential for physicians, therefore, to have a rational approach to the evaluation of a child or adolescent who presents to the ED with headache.

The purpose of this chapter is to review the etiologies, evaluation, appropriate investigations for nontraumatic headache and the available treatments in the ED or other acute settings in the pediatric population. The most common etiology of headache presenting to the ED is viral infections with fever. Migraine headache is one-fifth of these referrals: 18–21%. This chapter will review the available therapies for children, the guidelines that are used in pediatric headache centers and inpatient approaches if the headache is unresponsive to ED treatments.

6.1 Emergency-room evaluation and management

The initial evaluation of headaches should emphasize making the right diagnosis and differentiating primary from secondary headache before initiating any migraine therapy [2]. It is essential to keep in mind that, even if a patient has been diagnosed with migraine previously, they should still have a

Pediatric Headaches in Clinical Practice   Andrew D. Hershey, Paul Winner, Marielle A. Kabbouche and Scott W. Powers
© 2009 John Wiley & Sons, Ltd.

full evaluation to eliminate a possible secondary cause for the present headache.

Etiologies

Three studies have examined the chief complaint of headache in the ED. Burton *et al.* [3] reported that 1.3% of 53 988 visits to the Miami Children's Hospital ED during 1993 were for the evaluation of headache. The records of 288 children, approximately half of the children, were retrospectively reviewed. Serious neurologic diseases were found in 6.6% and included fifteen cases of viral meningitis, one shunt malfunction, one newly diagnosed hydrocephalus and one patient with lymphoma metastatic to the brain. Critically, all of these patients with serious neurologic conditions had abnormal findings on history or physical examination consistent with their diagnosis, except for a single patient with an unsuspected punctuate hemorrhage following head trauma.

Table 6.1   Spectrum of diagnoses for headache at Miami Children's Hospital ED 1993

Diagnosis	Amount (%)
Viral illness	39.2
Sinusitis	16
Migraine	15.6
Post-traumatic disorder	6.6
Viral meningitis	5.2
Streptococcal pharyngitis	4.9
Tension	4.5
Other	7.7

Adapted from Ref. [2].

A second study, from Barcelona, investigated 140 patients who warranted admission to a short-stay unit with an incoming diagnosis of headache [4]. Central nervous system tumors were found in six patients, five of whom had papilledema. The authors conclude that complete neurologic examination must be performed, leaving further 'complementary examinations for those cases where the patient history suggests organic alteration'. The third study retrospectively investigated the causes of acute headache in the pediatric ED and, similarly, found that viral infection with fever was the most common etiology [5]. Table 6.1 shows the most frequent diagnoses in this population of 150 consecutive children who presented with the abrupt evolution of headache.

Analysis of the clinical data revealed three important observations:

1. Only 2 of 150 children had occipital headache; both had posterior fossa tumors. Occipital location of the pain must be considered strongly indicative of an organic pathology, specifically posterior fossa tumors.

2. The majority of headaches in children and adolescents presenting to the ED are due to common conditions such as upper respiratory infection (URI) and migraine. These diagnoses are confirmed by history and physical examination.

3. In the three ED-based studies, all of the children with nontraumatic headache who had serious underlying conditions had demonstrable, objective findings on neurologic examination: alteration of consciousness, nuchal rigidity, papilledema, abnormal eye movements, ataxia or hemiparesis. Therefore, abnormality on neurologic examination is the principal indication for neuroimaging. The value of a normal neurologic examination cannot be stated too strongly.

Clinical approach to the child

The American College of Emergency Physicians issued a policy statement outlining the initial approach to adolescents presenting to the ED with a chief complaint of headache, excluding trauma-related headache. This document emphasizes a logical sequence of history and physical examination and appropriate laboratory or imaging studies and must be viewed as the standard of care for ED physicians.

Medical history

When evaluating a child with headache in the ED, the initial step is to gather history. The nature of the headache pain must be carefully addressed. Table 6.2 shows the key information that should be obtained for a medical history.

Physical and neurologic examination

Following this history, a thorough physical, neurologic examination (Table 6.3) and comprehensive headache examination (Table 6.4) must be conducted and include those elements shown in Tables 6.3 and 6.4.

Differential diagnosis

The most useful initial step in the development of a differential diagnosis is to categorize the headache into one of the five temporal patterns. The patterns seen commonly in the ED – acute, acute recurrent and chronic progressive – will be discussed below.

Table 6.2   Key information required from medical history

Temporal pattern or pace of onset of the headache
Acute, acute-recurrent, chronic progressive, chronic nonprogressive, or mixed
Duration
Frequency
Location

Quality and severity of pain
Associated symptoms, including nausea, vomiting, photophobia, phonophobia
Exacerbating/alleviating factors
Response to treatments
Aura

Past history of headache
Changing quality/location/severity of pain
Family history of headache
Toxic exposure

Drugs (prescribed or recreational)
Anticoagulants, anticonvulsants, birth control pills, asthma medicines, stimulants, anti-
   hypertensives, analgesics, carbon monoxide, lead
Trauma
Fever

Neurologic symptoms
Seizure, syncope, altered consciousness, declining school performance, neck pain or stiffness,
   vertigo, visual changes, diplopia, hearing loss or change, ataxia, disequilibrium, weakness,
   gait difficulty, back pain
Sinus or dental pain, nasal discharge, facial pain

Past medical history
Neurosurgical procedures (ventriculoperitoneal shunt)
Sinus disease
HIV
Endocrine disorders (hyperthyroidism)
Congenital heart disease (increased risk for brain abscess or hypertension)
Malignancy
Coagulopathy
Pregnancy and last menstrual period
Rheumatologic or collagen vascular disease (lupus)
Psychiatric disorders, such as depression, suicide, anxiety disorder

---

Table 6.3   Required elements of a thorough physical and neurologic examination

---

Vital signs
Blood pressure, pulse, respiration
General physical examination
Nuchal rigidity, Kernig and/or Brudzinski's sign, sinus, throat, temporomandibular joint,
 dental, cervical lymph node tenderness, ocular pressure, visual acuity, pain with eye
 movement, proptosis
Funduscopic examination
Papilledema, papillitis, retinal hemorrhage, venous pulsations
Cardiopulmonary examination
Skin rashes, petechiae, ecchymosis, needle tracts, neurocutaneous markers
Hepatosplenomegaly
Neurologic examination
Mental status: speech, orientation, alertness, behavior, changing level of consciousness
Cranial nerves: pupillary reaction, eye movements, facial movement
Motor: pronator drift, weakness, asymmetry
Coordination: dysmetria, intention tremor, rapid alternating movement
Deep tendon reflexes
Gait: tandem gait (tightrope walking) and station, Romberg's sign

---

The goal of an emergency room evaluation is to differentiate primary headaches from secondary headaches and act appropriately in ordering further necessary testing and specific therapies.

Acute headache

The causes of acute headaches presenting in the emergency room are listed in Table 6.5. The most common cause of acute headache in children is URI with fever.

Table 6.4   Comprehensive headache examination [6]. (Table based on information from Linder, *Pediatric Annals*, June 2005, Volume 34(6): 442–446)

---

1. Cervical spine examination
2. Skull: palpation of bones and muscles; listen for bruits
3. Ears: external auditory meatus occlusion and motion
4. Temporomandibular joint: palpation, range of motion
5. Nerves: palpation of supraorbital nerves, occipital nerves, examination of nerves IX through
   XII
6. Eyes: palpation, inspection
7. Sinuses: modified Muller maneuver
8. Evaluation of increased intracranial pressure
9. Teeth: inspection, percussion, palpation

Table 6.5 Causes of acute headache

Paranasal infection	Hypertension
URI with fever	Trauma
Sinusitis	Substance abuse
Otitis	Cocaine
Pharyngitis	Medications
Meningitis	Intoxications
Subarachnoid hemorrhage	Carbon monoxide
Intracranial hemorrhage	Lead
Migraine	Hypertension

The presence of headache plus fever, however, must raise concerns for meningitis, either bacterial or viral. If clinical examination demonstrates nuchal rigidity without alteration of consciousness, signs of increased intracranial pressure or lateralizing features, then lumbar puncture is mandatory. If the mental status is altered or focal findings evident, then cranial imaging is warranted prior to lumbar puncture, though blood cultures should be drawn and antibiotics empirically begun before the patient is transported for neuroimaging.

Another common, although overdiagnosed, cause for headache with fever is sinusitis and represents 9 to 16% of the causes of headache in the ED in children. If clinical history and physical examinations suggest acute sinusitis, then sinus X-ray films or computed tomography (CT) scans of the sinuses are indicated.

Headache with or without fever in a patient with human immunodeficiency virus (HIV) infection, or other immuno-compromised state, requires an aggressive investigation for opportunistic central nervous system (CNS) infection, such as toxoplasmosis, cytomegalovirus (CMV), herpes simplex virus (HSV), fungi, atypical tuberculosis or CNS lymphoma.

If history suggests a sudden, severe ('thunderclap') onset to the headache, then subarachnoid hemorrhage (SAH) must be considered. SAH is rare in children and has three primary causes: (1) arteriovenous malformation (AVM) (cavernous angioma, venous angioma, capillary telangiectasia and true AVM); (2) aneurysm (berry, giant, traumatic and mycotic); and (3) miscellaneous causes, including coagulopathy, sickle cell anemia, sympathomimetic intoxication and leukemia.

A noncontrasted head CT is warranted in those patients with suspected SAH. Small bleeds may be difficult to detect, in which case lumbar puncture must be conducted. Comparison of the red cell count and supernatant between tubes 1 and 4 may be useful in the distinction of traumatic spinal tap from the hemorrhagic cerebrospinal fluid (CSF) of SAH. Coagulation studies and platelet counts must be checked.

A patient with a prior neurosurgical procedure, such as ventriculo- perito-neal shunt placement, who develops headache must raise concerns for the possibility of shunt malfunction, with or without infection. Should the history suggest potential exposure to carbon monoxide, then the carboxy-hemoglobin level needs to be evaluated and the patient given 100% oxygen.

The overwhelming majority of acute headaches in children and adolescents are due to common conditions such as URI with fever or migraine headache. These diagnoses are established by medical history and thorough physical and neurologic examination. In the three pediatric ED-based studies discussed earlier, all patients presenting with nontraumatic headache who were found to have serious underlying conditions had objective neurologic findings such as alteration of consciousness, nuchal rigidity, papilledema, abnormal eye move-ments, ataxia or hemiparesis. Therefore, abnormality on neurologic examina-tion is the principal indication for neuroimaging. The value of a normal neurologic examination cannot be overstated.

Chronic progressive headache

This temporal pattern describes headaches that gradually increase in frequency and severity over time. This is the most ominous of the five temporal profiles and carries with it the greatest likelihood of organic pathology. The differential diagnosis of chronic progressive headache is listed in Table 6.6.

When this pattern of headache is accompanied by symptoms and signs of increased intracranial pressure, an aggressive evaluation for space-occupying lesions must be conducted. Several associated historic clues may further heighten the chances of tumor, abscess, hematoma or vascular anomaly.

Table 6.6 Chronic progressive headache

Hydrocephalus	Cryptococcal
Obstructive	Lyme disease
Communicating	Pseudotumor cerebri
Neoplasm	Aneurysm
Medulloblastoma	Malformations
Cerebellar astrocytoma	Chiari
Ependymoma	Dandy–Walker
Pineal-region tumor	Hypertension
Craniopharyngioma	Medications
Astrocytoma	Birth control pills
Brain abscess	Stimulants
Subdural hematoma	Intoxications
Chronic meningitis	Carbon monoxide
	Lead poisoning

Morning headache or headaches that awaken the child from sleep are classic symptoms of the dependent edema of intracranial lesions and obstructive hydrocephalus. Likewise, nocturnal or morning emesis, with or without headache, suggest increased intracranial pressure and are particularly common symptoms of tumors arising near the floor of the fourth ventricle. Between headaches, behavioral or mood changes, some of which may be subtle, are described by parents. Cognitive changes (demonstrated by declining school performance) can, on occasion, be the presenting complaint. Careful history can ferret out these associated features. There is no invariable brain tumor headache profile. It is essential to recognize this temporal pattern of escalating headache frequency and severity that then dictates a course of action. An MRI scan is much more useful than a CT scan in this setting, since it permits better visualization and definition of an intracranial structural abnormality.

In 1991, the findings of The Childhood Brain Tumor Consortium study were reported [7]. Detailed analysis of over 3000 children with brain tumors demonstrated that 98% had at least one of five sign, including papilledema, ataxia, hemiparesis, abnormal eye movements or depressed reflexes. Some 50% of the patients had five signs at diagnosis.

Five key points on neurologic examination must be documented when assessing a child with chronic progressive headache: (1) optic discs, (2) eye movements, (3) pronator drift, (4) tandem gait and (5) deep tendon reflexes (DTRs). Papilledema may be difficult to appreciate in the young or uncooperative child. Even in experienced hands, direct ophthalmoscopy can be a challenge.

Acute recurrent headaches

This pattern of headache implies episodes of headache separated by symptom free intervals (Table 6.7). The vast majority of acute recurrent headaches in children and adolescents are either migraine or tension-type headaches. Although there is some controversy as to which of these two is the most frequent, few would argue that the two represent the majority of episodic headaches.

Table 6.7 Causes of acute recurrent headache

Migraine
Migraine variants
Tension-type
Cluster
Neuralgias
Hypertension
Medications

6.2 Treatments of primary headache in a pediatric emergency room

Treating an acute episode in children and adolescents has been a challenge in the emergency room due to the lack of guidelines and standardization of available medications. Therapeutic approaches vary from one emergency room to another. Multiple studies reveal that polypharmacology is used in 82%; more than three medications are used in 25%. Available specific treatments for migraine headache in an emergency-room setting include the following: antidopaminergic medications such as prochlorperazine and metoclopramide; nonsteroidal anti-inflammatory drugs (NSAIDs): ketorolac, dihydroergotamine (DHE); antiepileptic drugs: sodium valproate and triptan (Figure 6.1).

Antidopaminergic drugs: (prochlorperazine and metoclopramide)

The use of these medications is not limited to control the nausea and vomiting often present during a migraine headache. Their use is aimed at their antidopamine effect to abort an underlying pathological process involving the dopaminergic system during a migraine attack. Prochlorperazine has been shown to be very effective in aborting an attack in the emergency room when given intravenously with a load of intravenous fluid. Results show a 75% improvement with 50% headache freedom at 1 h and 95% improvement with 60% headache freedom at 3 h [8]. When prochlorperazine was compared with metoclopramide and placebo in a randomized prospective double blinded placebo-controlled study, the response to prochlorperazine was 82% improvement in headache severity, 42% response with metoclopramide and 29% with placebo [9]. These results show that metoclopramide and prochlorperazine are both effective in migraine treatment compared with placebo but that

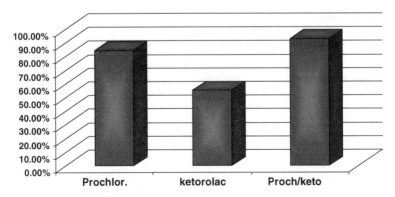

Figure 6.1 Acute therapy for primary headache in the pediatric emergency room.

Table 6.8   Randomized prospective double-blinded placebo-controlled study [9]. (Table based on information from Coppola *et al.*, *Ann Emerg Med*, April 1996)

	Prochlorperazine	Metoclopramide	Placebo
Pain improvement (%)	82	46	29

prochlorperazine has a higher response. The average dose of metoclopramide uses is 0.13–0.15 mg/kg with a maximum dose of 10 mg given intravenously over 15 min.

The average dose of prochlorperazine is 0.15 mg/kg with a maximum dose of 10 mg. These medications are usually well tolerated, but extrapyramidal reactions are more frequent in children than in the older population. An acute extrapyramidal reaction can be controlled in the emergency room with 25–50 mg of diphenhydramine given intravenously (Table 6.8).

The effectiveness of prochlorperazine in aborting intractable migraine in children was also retrospectively reviewed at Cincinnati Children's Hospital Medical Center [8]: 20 patients, known migraineurs, were tabulated and their ED charts reviewed. These patients were diagnosed by International Headache Society criteria in the headache center and referred to the ED at one point for treatment for acute intractable headache.

The mean headache severity was 8.4 on admission to the ED, the mean headache duration was 54 h and the mean prochlorperazine dose was 0.13 mg/kg.

A 75% improvement was seen at 1 h with 50% headache freedom. A 95% improvement was seen at 3 h with 60% headache freedom. Headache was considered better if there was a noticeable improvement of more than 50% from baseline.

NSAIDs: ketorolac

It is known that an aseptic inflammation occurs in the central nervous system due to the effect of multiple reactive peptides. Outpatient treatment with over-the-counter anti-inflammatory medications is effective and widespread. Ketorolac is often used in the ED as monotherapy for a migraine attack or in combination with other drugs. In monotherapy, the response to ketorolac is 55.2% improvement. When combined with prochlorperazine, the response rate jumps to 93%. Recurrence rate in 24 h when ketorolac is used is 30% [10, 11]. The explanation of such a high rate of recurrence may be due to the use of ketorolac in patients with an analgesic rebound headache.

These patients have been overusing their outpatient abortive treatment, including their NSAIDs. Ketorolac in these cases will only bring a temporary relief. These patients would probably benefit more from other migraine treatment, including sodium valproate and/or DHE (Figure 6.2).

Antiepileptic drugs: sodium valproate

Antiepileptic drugs have been used as a prophylactic treatment for migraine headache for years with adequate double-blinded controlled studies on their efficacy in adults [12–15].

Studies for use of sodium valproate in children and adolescents are currently underway.

Sodium valproate has been introduced in children recently as an abortive treatment for acute attacks with promising response. The mechanism in which sodium valproate acutely aborts migraine headaches is not well understood. Sodium valproate is given as a bolus of 15–20 mg/kg push over 5 min [13–16]. This intravenous load is to be followed by an oral dose (15–20 mg/day) in the 4 h after the injection. Patients may benefit from a short-term preventive treatment with an extended release form after discharge from the emergency room. Sodium valproate is usually well tolerated. Patients should be receiving a fluid load during the procedure. Studies for use of other anticonvulsant drugs have been inconclusive and soon will be repeated.

Triptan

Linder [17], in an open-label study, documented the effectiveness of subcutaneous sumatriptan 0.06 mg/kg and showed an overall efficacy of 72% at 30 min and 78% at 2 h, with a recurrence rate of 6%. Because children tend to have a shorter duration of headache, a recurrence rate of 6% would seem appropriate for this population.

DHE, if recommended for the recurrences, should not be given in the 24 h of the triptan use.

DHE

DHE is an old migraine medication used as a vasoconstrictor to abort the vascular phase of migraine headache. The effectiveness will be discussed in detail in the inpatient treatment of migraine. One dose of DHE can be effective in the ED. When compared with the sodium valproate the response was as follows [15]:

	1 h	2 h	4 h	24 h	Side effects
Valproate (%)	50	60	60	60	0
DHE with metoclopramide (%)	45	50	60	90	15

Effectiveness of approaches mentioned in treatment of acute intractable migraine in children and adolescents

Studies are limited, but the reviews available show an acceptable outcome at 48–72 h with a recurrence rate of 29%, which includes the 6% who need a more prolonged inpatient treatment.

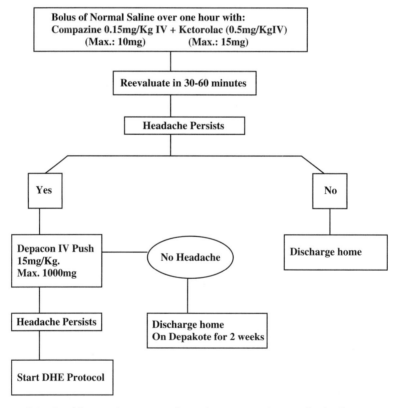

Figure 6.2 Prochlorperazine versus ketorolac prospective randomized double-blind study [11] consisting of 62 children, 5–18 years of age: ketorolac (used at 0.5 mg/kg; max. 30 mg) or intravenous prochlorperazine (at 0.15 mg/kg). At 1 h: 84.8% response to prochloroperazine; 55.2% response to ketorolac; 93% response when treatments were combined; 30% recurrence. (Figure based on information published in *Ann Emerg Med*, Vol 43, Brousseau *et al.*, 'Treatment of pediatric migraine headaches: a randomized double blind trial of prochlorperazine versus ketorolac' © Elsevier 2004)

6.3 Management of primary headache in an inpatient unit

Some 6–7% of patients fail acute treatment in the ED. These patients are usually admitted for a 3–5-day stay and receive extensive parenteral treatment. A child should be admitted to the hospital for a primary headache when they: (1) are status migrainous; (2) have an exacerbation of chronic severe headache; or (3) are in an analgesic rebound headache.

The goal of inpatient treatment is to control a disabling headache that has been unresponsive to other abortive therapy and is disabling to the child. Treatment protocols include the use of DHE, antiemetics, sodium valproate and others.

DHE

Ergots are one of the oldest treatments for migraine headache. DHE is a parenteral form used for acute exacerbations. Its effect is due to the 5HT1A-1B-1D-1F receptor agonist affinity and central vasoconstriction. DHE has a greater alpha adrenergic antagonist activity and is less vasoconstrictive peripherally. Two pediatric protocols are recommended in children and adolescents. The first one uses more frequent injections but lower doses to prevent side effects; the second protocol is more aggressive and uses higher doses for a faster response.

Before initiation of these protocols, a full history and neurological examination should be obtained. Girls of child-bearing age should be evaluated for any concerns for pregnancy.

Low-dose DHE

In the low-dose protocol [18], DHE is administered with metoclopramide to prevent gastroenteral side effects including nausea vomiting and abdominal discomfort. The dose of DHE varies with patient age. The following protocol is used:

Age (years)	Metoclopramide (mg/dose)	DHE/dose (mg/dose)
6–9	5–10	0.1
9–12	5–10	0.15
12–16	5–10	0.2

For metoclopramide at a dose of 0.2 mg/kg, a maximum of 10 mg is given 0.5 h prior to the administration of the DHE. DHE is repeated every 6 h for a maximum of 16 doses.

When headache ceases, give an extra dose to prevent recurrence. DHE dose may be increased by 0.05 mg/dose until abdominal discomfort.

High-dose DHE protocol

In the high-dose protocol [19], patients are premedicated with 0.13–0.15 mg/kg of prochlorperazine 0.5 h prior to the DHE dose. A dose of 0.5–1 mg (depending on age and tolerability) is used every 8 h until headache freedom. When headache ceases, an extra dose is given. After three doses, the prochlorperazine is replaced by a different antiemetic to prevent extrapyramidal reactions. The response to this protocol is a 97% improvement and 77% headache freedom. The response starts being noticeable by dose 5 and can reach its maximum effect after dose 10 (Figure 6.3). Side effects of DHE include nausea, vomiting, abdominal discomfort, flushed face and increased blood pressure. During the hospital admission the patient is usually started on migraine prophylaxis, depending on the patient's history and comorbid problems.

Sodium valproate

Sodium valproate is used when DHE is contraindicated or has been ineffective. One adult study recommends the use of sodium valproate as follows [16]: bolus with 15 mg/kg then follow with 5 mg/kg every 8 h until headache freedom or up to 10 doses, whichever comes first. Always give an extra dose after headache ceases. This protocol was studied in adults with chronic daily headaches and

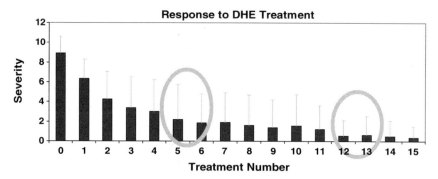

Figure 6.3 Response to high-dose DHE protocol. The main response to the protocol is noticeable by the fifth dose; patients may complain of worsening of their headache with the first two or three doses before noticing an improvement. If the pain is improving, then the DHE should be continued until headache freedom with a maximum of 15–20 doses, due to the curve dip that is seen by the dose 12. If *no* improvement at all is noticed by the fifth or sixth dose, then another acute therapy should be considered, such as sodium valproate.

showed an 80% improvement. Sodium valproate reveals a new perspective in childhood headache. It is well tolerated and is useful when DHE is contra-indicated or not tolerated.

6.4 Conclusions

The majority of headaches during childhood and adolescence presenting to the ED are caused by self-limited illnesses or medically remediable conditions.

Serious disorders, such as tumors, meningitis, hemorrhages or abscesses, are infrequent and, when present, are accompanied by objective neurologic signs.

The most important neuron-diagnostic tool in the evaluation of headache in children is a *careful history and detailed neurological examination*. Exploration of the onset, pace and evolution of the symptom complex will dictate the scope and urgency of ancillary testing.

Primary headaches can frequently be debilitating. Aggressive management may prevent severe disability and failure at school if initiated early. It is imperative to state that treatments available for use for acute migraine headache in children and adolescents are off-label. Their use is widespread, but double-blind placebo-controlled studies are still unavailable for this age group.

References

1. Rassmussen, B.K., Jensen, R., Schroll, M. *et al.* (1991) Epidemiology of headache in a general population – a prevalance study. *Journal of Clinical Epidemiology*, **44**, 1147–1157.
2. Lewis, D.W. and Qureshi, F.A. (2000) Acute headache in the pediatric emergency department. *Headache*, **40**, 200–203.
3. Burton, L.J., Quinn, B., Pratt-Cheney, J.L. *et al.* (1997) Headache etiology in a pediatric emergency room. *Pediatric Emergency Care*, **13**, 1–4.
4. Lobera Gutiérrez de Pando, E., Lopez Navarro, J.A., Youssef Fasheh, W. *et al.* (1999) Headache in a short-stay unit. A retrospective study of 140 cases. *Anales Espanoles de PediatrÚa*, **50**(6), 562–565 (in Spanish).
5. Kan, L., Nagelberg, J. and Maytal, J. (2000) Headaches in a pediatric emergency department: etiology, imaging and treatment. *Headache*, **40**(1), 25–29.
6. Linder, S. (2005) Understanding the comprehensive pediatric headache examination. *Pediatric Annals*, **34**(6), 442–446.
7. The Childhood Brain Tumor Consortium (1991) The epidemiology of headache among children with brain tumors. Headache in children with brain tumors. *Journal of Neuro-Oncology*, **10**, 31–46.

8. Kabbouche, M.A., Vockell, A.l., LeCates, S.L. *et al.* (2001) Tolerability and effectiveness of prochlorperazine for intractable migraine. *Pediatrics*, **107**(4), E62.

9. Coppola, M., Yealy, D.M. and Leibold, R.A. (1995) Randomized placebo-controlled evaluation of prochlorperazine versus metoclopramide for emergency department treatment of migraine headache. *Annals of Emergency Medicine*, **26**(5), 541–546.

10. Larkin, G. (1999) Intravenous ketorolac vs intravenous prochlorperazine for the treatment of migraine headaches. *Academic Emergency Medicine*, **6**, 668–670.

11. Brousseau, D.C., Duffy, S.J., Anderson, A.C. and Linakis, J.G. (2004) Treatment of pediatric migraine headaches: a randomized, double-blind trial of prochlorperazine versus ketorolac. *Annals of Emergency Medicine*, **43**(2), 256–262.

12. Freitag, G. Collins, S.D., Carlson, H.A. *et al.* (2002) A randomized trial of divalproex sodium extended-release tablets in migraine prophylaxis. *Neurology*, **58**(11), 1652–1659.

13. Mathew, N.T., Kailasam, J., Meadors, L. *et al.* (2000) Intravenous valproate sodium (Depacon) aborts migraine rapidly: a preliminary report. *Headache*, **40**(9), 720–723.

14. Tanen, D.A., Miller, S., French, T. and Riffenburgh, R.H. (2003) Intravenous sodium valproate versus prochlorperazine for the emergency department of acute treatment of acute migraine headaches; a prospective, randomized, double-blind trial. *Annals of Emergency Medicine*, **41**(6), 847–853.

15. Edwards, K.R., Norton, J. and Behnke, M. (2001) Comparison of intravenous valproate versus intramuscular dihydroergotamine and metoclopramide for acute migraine headache. *Headache*, **41**, 976–980.

16. Schwatz, T.H., Kapritskiy, V.V. and Sohn, R.S. (2002) Intraveinous valproate sodium in the treatment of daily headache. *Headache*, **42**(6), 519–522.

17. Linder, S.L. (1996) Subcutaneous sumatriptan in the clinical setting: the first 50 consecutive patients with acute migraine in a pediatric neurology office practice. *Headache*, **36**, 419–422.

18. Linder, S.L. (1994) Treatment of acute childhood migraine headache with dihydroergotamine mesylate. *Headache*, **34**, 578–580.

19. Kabbouche, M.A., Powers, S.W., Vockell, A.B. *et al.* (2003) Inpatient management of pediatric patients for intractable headache and status migrainosus. *Headache*, **42**, 551.

7
Pathophysiology of primary headaches

Andrew D. Hershey

An understanding of the etiology of the primary headache disorders is beginning to be elucidated. By their very definition, primary headaches are due to an intrinsic problem with the brain or nervous system. A variety of approaches can be used to attempt to understand the pathophysiology, and in recent years this has included neuroimaging, neurophysiology, and genetics and molecular biology. Many of the pathophysiological components appear to have overlaps between the various primary headache disorders. The majority of the research has been focused on migraine, with some advances being made in tension-type headaches (TTHs) and trigeminal autonomic cephalalgias. In the latter, the naming of these headaches as trigeminal autonomic celphalalgias directly implies the involvement of both the trigeminal cranial nerve and the sympathetic and parasympathetic nervous system. Several detailed reviews have been written recently that address many of these pathophysiological models in more detail and should be reviewed for a more in-depth understanding of the mechanisms.

7.1 Migraine

Migraine has been one of the major areas for an understanding of the biological basis of primary headaches. Broadly speaking, the pathophysiology of migraine has evolved from a vascular model to more of a neurological disease with a vascular reaction (the neurovascular model or trigeminal vascular model). This

Pediatric Headaches in Clinical Practice   Andrew D. Hershey, Paul Winner, Marielle A. Kabbouche and Scott W. Powers
© 2009 John Wiley & Sons, Ltd.

evolution to a neurological basis for migraine has been made through the recognition of the role of inheritance and molecular biomarkers that are beginning to be discovered. The mechanism of triggering a migraine is likely due to an inherited propensity that allows common environmental changes – both intrinsic (i.e. hormonal, skipping meals, change in sleep patterns) and extrinsic (i.e. whether changes, motion sickness) – to start a cascade of biological processes that ultimately results in the neurological and vascular changes that result in a migraine.

7.1.1 Genetic factors

Patients have long noted that headaches 'run in the family'. This observation by families has been consistent over time and identifies the underlying genetic nature of primary headaches and implies an underlying genetic disorder. Whereas the variation within families reveals the variable expression combined with environmental influences, the variation across families and individuals argues for a polygenetic nature of migraine. For pediatric headache, the presence of a strong family history of headaches is often observed and has been suggested as part of the criteria for the diagnosis of migraine [1].

The genetic basis of primary headache and migraine has the potential for identifying the underlying molecular basis of primary headache disorders. This potential is the greatest for migraine, where several genes have begun to be identified for rare migraine subtypes, while population and twin studies confirm this genetic basis. Given the wide heterogeneity of migraine and primary headache disorders, there are most likely multiple genes involved in the pathogenesis and phenotypic expression of migraine and other primary headache disorders.

7.1.2 Population studies

The use of population-based studies for potential genetic disease relies on the coassociation of the disease within families and often includes twin studies. For migraine, this is complicated by the high prevalence rate of migraine in the general population. This high prevalence rate increases the chance occurrence within a family and, thus, increases the familial associations.

In order to address some of these issues, Russell et al. [2] investigated a sample of 4000 individuals from the Danish Central Persons Registry. All people within this registry exclusively with migraine with aura and a random, equivalent number of people exclusively with migraine without aura were selected to be studied (probands). All probands that participated in the telephone interviews, along with their spouses and first-degree relatives over 18, were included. Comparing both familial and spousal occurrence of migraine, it was found that for migraines without aura there was a 1.9-fold increased familial risk of having migraine without aura, whereas unrelated spouses had a 1.5-fold increased risk. This suggested that there were both genetic and environmental contributions for migraine without aura. This was even greater for migraine with aura, with first-degree relatives having a fourfold increased risk of migraine with aura, whereas spouses showed no increase. Russell [3] went on to review this study, along with other reported genetic studies, and identified that the population relative risk for migraine without aura ranged from 1.44 to 3.09, depending on the generation assessed. This risk was greatest in children of parents with migraine without aura, with a 3.43-fold increased risk, although only adult children were assessed. The population relative risk was even higher for migraine with aura, ranging from 2.68 to as high as 4.85. The onset of migraine with aura had the greatest relative risk of being inherited if the proband developed their migraine in the teen years. He also reviewed the various inheritance patterns. These have included both autosomal dominant and autosomal recessive inheritance patterns, as well as polygenic and 'sex-linked' patterns. This same review examined the inheritance pattern of cluster headaches, noting even higher population relative risk (up to 62.8 in a study by Kudrow and Kudrow [4]).

Population twin studies

Twin-based population studies, comparing monozygotic twins with same-sex dizygotic twins can help separate the genetic from the environmental contributions. In the population-based New Danish Twin Register of 2026 monozygotic twins and 3334 same-sex dizygotic twins, the prevalence rate for twins was similar to the population rate [5]. In the follow-up to this study [6], proband comparison was performed and the pairwise concordance rate was found to be much higher for monozygotic twins (28%) compared with same-sex dizygotic twins (18%), while a probandwise comparison was even higher (40% vesus 28% respectively). This study clearly identified a genetic factor in migraine; however, the lack of complete agreement (i.e. 100% comparison) identifies the complexity in the migraine inheritance pattern.

A population-based twin study of children, aged 8 to 9 years old, from Sweden was studied using the International Classification of Headache Disorders(ICHD-I) criteria [7]. Of those children who reported having had headaches, 79% of them were classified as migraine or TTHs. The study found that a probandwise concordance was highest for monozygotic girls and boys at 0.52 and 0.51 respectively, although same-sex dizygotic boys and girls were intermediate at 0.22 and 0.27 respectively, whereas the concordance rate was 0.15 for opposite-sex dizygotic children. This was for all headache types; when the headaches were divided into migraine, TTHs and unclassified headaches, the concordance for monozygotic twins was higher than for dizygotic twins for all subgroups, although the numbers were small for a large-scale conclusion. This analysis did demonstrate, however, that there was a positive inheritance pattern for both migraine and TTHs, with migraine headaches being greater.

Population family studies

The genetic basis of migraine can also be addressed using a family-based method. Kallela and coworkers [8, 9] examined the co-occurrence of migraine without aura and migraine with aura within families using a standardized, validated questionnaire. This study examined three potential familial patterns for migraine: migraine with aura but not migraine without aura; migraine without aura and migraine with aura; or a combination of both migraine with aura and migraine without aura. Of this group of 210 families, or 906 individuals, that could differentiate their migraine type, 11.3% had experienced migraine with aura, 23.8% experienced migraine without aura, and 41.2% had a combination of both. In addition, 3.2% had aura without headache, while 20.5% had unclassifiable aura by ICHD-I criteria. They further observed that, if the patients had a combination of migraine with aura and migraine without aura, they were more likely to have severe headaches and were, therefore, more likely to be seen in a subspecialty clinic. This is in contrast to the general population distribution of migraine without aura and migraine with aura, suggesting again that the aura contributes a higher degree of inheritance.

Stewart et al. [10] evaluated the characteristics of the proband on the familial risk of migraine. First-degree relative of 532 individuals with migraines were compared with controlled subjects. The relative risk of migraine in first-degree relatives was increased to 1.88, similar to that reported by Russell et al. [2]. When migraine characteristics were analyzed in the proband and the relative risk of migraine in the first-degree relative compared with controls, they found that the relative risk was increased in the first-degree relatives if the onset of migraine in the proband was prior to age 16 years (relative risk 2.50), if the severity was described as typically 9–10 on a 10-point scale (relative risk 2.38), or if the proband had migraine with aura (relative risk 2.19). The observation of early age of onset and increased relative risk reaffirms the clinical observation/criteria of Prensky of assisting with the diagnosis of migraine in children [1] and stresses the importance of a familial component in the diagnosis and management of pediatric migraine.

Environmental influences

A major limitation for many of these population-based studies is the balance between the genetic influence and the environmental influence. To address this limitation, Gervil *et al.* [11] compared the concordance rate in monozygotic and dizygotic twins using a model assessing the genetic and environmental contributions. Testing a variety of models, including an additive model, shared model, nonshared model and nonadditive model, they found the additive genetics model to obtain a best fit for the contribution of genetics and environment to migraine without aura. In this model, genetics contributed 61% and the environment contributed 39%. In this concept, the genetic potential served as the basis for development of migraine, while an additional environmental contribution was necessary for the expression.

Gervil and coworkers refined this in a study of 169 discordant twins (i.e. one twin with migraine with aura the other without migraine), comparing possible environmental risk factors [12]. This study failed to identify any specific environmental risk factors, in contrast to other diseases examined with this registry. They did note that most of the twins were raised in the same household, so environmental factors would only diverge during adulthood and that adoption-based studies may be needed to identify true environmental factors.

For the other primary headache disorders, the genetic contributions are less clear. On the Danish twin study, the contribution of environment was much more notable for TTH (81%) than genetics (19%), making the likelihood of TTH being an inheritable disorder low [13]. For cluster headache, there appears to be two forms based on some of the molecular genetics described below: a familial form and a spontaneous form.

7.1.3 Specific genes

Individual genes and polymorphism identification

In contrast to population genetics, molecular biology genetics attempts to identify the particular genes responsible for migraine and primary headache disorders. Although predominantly focused on migraine, this also includes identification of potential cluster headache genetic identification. The identification of specific polymorphisms has focused on familial hemiplegic migraine with three genes identified. Multiple other genes, however, have also been implicated into the pathophysiology of migraine, including channels, mitochondrial genome, serotonin genome, dopamine genome, thrombotic and vascular risk factors, and inflammation. Several reviews have examined these potential etiologies [14–16].

Familial hemiplegic migraine: CACNA1A

In this migraine subtype there is a distinct inheritance of migraines, where the migraines are associated with hemiplegia. Multiple pedigrees have been examined, and in 1993 Joutel et al. [17] identified a linkage of familial hemiplegic migraine to chromosome 19. This was confirmed by Terwindt et al. [18], while also observing that some of the families were not linked to this locus. In 1996, Ophoff et al. [19] identified that this linkage to chromosome 19p13 was due to mutations in the brain-specific P/Q-type calcium channel α1-subunit (CACN-L1A4; later, the nomenclature was changed to CACNA1A). Not only do mutations in this channel contribute to hemiplegic migraine, but they are also noted to be associated with episodic ataxia type 2.

With the identification of alterations in this P/Q-type calcium channel, further studies have identified both variable clinical expression of the mutations [20] and genetic heterogeneity within families [21] with a broad spectrum of presentations. This clinical spectrum varied across attacks with some that are coassociated with coma and prolonged hemiplegia, while others may be associated with nystagmus and ataxia. Given the coassociation of this chain with episodic ataxia type 2, this overlapping spectrum suggests that the interplay and variable expression within this channelopathy may contribute to both disorders.

Familial hemiplegic migraine: ATP1A2

The discovery of the P/Q-type calcium channel as a contributor to familial hemiplegic migraine identified a significant contribution of genetics to the pathophysiology of this disorder; however, it was not identified in all family pedigrees with this disorder. Subsequent chromosomal mapping and linkage analysis identified an additional locus on chromosome 1q31 [22] and chromosome 1q23 [23]. In 2003, De Fusco et al. [24] identified that the gene affected was the α2 subunit of the Na$^+$/K$^+$ pump (ATP1A2). The product of this gene was localized not at the synapse, but rather in the astrocytes surrounding the nerve endings and connecting to the blood vessels. This suggested that the influence of this gene was due to energy stabilization at the synapse with neurotransmission altered at the synapse by the milieu in which the synapse was located (reviewed by Moskowitz *et al.* [25]).

As with the CACNA1A gene, multiple mutations and polymorphisms have been identified and association with other disease states identified. The variability of the mutations also appears to have variable characteristics [26]. The polymorphisms in this gene have also been associated with benign familial infantile convulsions [27] and alternating hemiplegia of childhood [28]. In addition to familial hemiplegic migraine, a single mutation in the ATP1A2 gene has also been identified in a family with basilar-type migraine, suggesting an additional overlap with these migraine subtypes.

Familial hemiplegic migraine: SCN1A

A third gene has recently been identified to be associated with this disorder by Dichgans *et al.* [29]. This gene was found to be located on chromosome 2q24 and encoded a neuronal voltage-gated sodium channel (SCN1A). Electrophysiology of this genetic defect revealed that recordings of cells transfected with this defective channel had accelerated recovery in fast inactivation, suggesting a more rapid response in these channels and possibly contributing to the hypersensitivity seen in migraine pathophysiology.

Other gene contributions

Within the last few years, several additional genetic and biological markers for migraines have been postulated in both children and adults. The significance and widespread applicability of these genetic polymorphisms and biomarkers are yet to be identified, but may help in a more clear understanding of the basis type of physiology.

Serotonin

The role of serotonin in migraines has been long implicated in the pathophysiology and treatment options. Studies have also shown that, during a migraine, there are altered levels of serotonin in the blood [30]. Serotonin levels will fall during a migraine, with corresponding administration of serotonin relieving the attack. Platelets have been implicated as modulating levels of serotonin, and some of the neurological changes seen during a migraine have been attributed to this alteration. The changes in the levels of serotonin, however, are small and the serotonin effect may be from a central activation of serotonin receptors [31]; that is, changes in serotonin receptors within the brain [32]. These changes in central 5-HT receptors may be contribute to the increased hypersensitivity that occurs in migraineurs [33, 34] and to the decreased habituation to external stimuli [35, 36] and may be the basis for trigeminal nociception [37, 38].

Polymorphisms in the serotonin transporter gene (5HTTLPR) were identified, with two polymorphic regions noted: one with a short base-pair region of 484 base pairs and one with a long base-pair region of 528 polymorphisms [39]. Patients with migraine were compared with controls and could be classified as having two short regions, two long regions, or a mixture. In this study, there was no difference between migraineurs and controls. However, within migraineur patients with the short–short genotype had an increased frequency of attacks. Thus, this gene could be viewed not as a genetic cause, but as a genetic modifier.

Borroni *et al.* [40] extended this observation by comparing subjects that had migraine with aura with subjects that had migraine without aura. In this comparison, subjects that had migraine with aura were much more likely to have the short–short genotype than did subjects that had migraine without aura or controls (increased odds ratios of 2.60 and 2.14 respectively).

The contribution of the serotonin transporter gene polymorphisms in pediatric migraine was examined by Szilagyi *et al.* [41]. In this study, not only was the above polymorphism studied (5-HTTLPR), but a second polymorphism within the second intron (STin2) was also noted to have variable-length repeat units. No differences were noted in the comparison of 87 children with migraine versus 464 controls without migraine in either of the 5HTTLPR or STin2 polymorphisms. When subgroup analysis was performed, they found differential expression of the STin2 genotype that was homozygous for the longer polymorphism (12 repeats) compared with the heterozygotic or the shorter unit (10 repeats) states. The longer polymorphism was associated not only with an increased risk of migraine with aura, but also with increased vomiting and abdominal pain. This was limited to 38 children with migraine with aura and 41 children with significant abdominal symptoms, and the increased expression was only noted in 52.6% and 58.5% respectively compared with a control level of 37.1%. Further phenotypic and genotypic characterization needs to be performed on larger population; however, it is intriguing that this polymorphism may serve as both a genetic basis of aura and as a disease modifier for abdominal symptoms.

Potassium channel

The identification of familial hemiplegic migraine as channelopathy has lead to investigation of additional channels. Mössner *et al.* evaluated the poly-glutamine region of the KCNN3 potassium channel as a potential candidate for migraines [42]. In their study, 190 patients were compared to 232 controls for variation in this highly polymorphic region. This region of the KCNN3 gene has variable numbers of CAG repeats ranging from 12 to 24. In this region, the genotype with 15 repeats was more common in migraine without aura and migraine with aura than with controls. Although this was statistically signifi-cant, it was also one of the lowest number of patients or controls, thus the applicability of the observation may be limited. Although this does not describe a pathophysiological nature of why this repeats contribute to this disorder, it again supports the possible channel involvement.

5′,10′-Methylenetetrahydrofolate reductase (MTHFR)

5′,10′-Methylenetetrahydrofolate reductase is a key enzyme involved with metabolism of folate. A common polymorphism in this gene is C677T, which changes an alanine to a valine at position 222. In the homozygote state for valine, there is an increased plasma total homocystine level and, thus, a possible increased stroke risk. In a study by Scher *et al.*, [43] adults with migraine with aura, migraine without aura, and nonmigraineurs were compared for the presence of this polymorphism. This study found that patients with migraine with aura had an increased odds ratio of 2.05 of having the homozygote valine genotype, while the odds ratio of migraine without aura was decreased (0.77, not significant) compared with controls. This may provide a biomarker for further studies of migraine with aura compared with migraine without aura and controls.

Hypocretin receptor 2 (HCRTR2)

In two studies on the genetics of cluster headaches, polymorphisms in the HCRTR2 gene were analyzed. This receptor is located in the posterolateral hypothalamus and regulates the sleep–wake cycle. In a study by Schürks *et al.* [44], having the G1246A polymorphism in this gene increases the odds ratio of having cluster headaches to 1.97 compared with controls. On the other hand, in a study by Baumber *et al.* [45] evaluating sporadic cluster headaches, no association was seen. This conflicting data suggests that the familial hemiplegic migraine may have a genetic component, whereas the sporadic component would be more difficult to identify as the genetic association.

Microarray genomics

Molecular biology can also be used to identify potential pathways of activation during a disease state, as well as allow for screening of large expression-level changes. Microarray genomic analysis is one such method. In this method, RNA can be isolated from whole blood cells and examined for overall expression of a variety of genes with the whole human genome analyzed at one period. We have demonstrated that distinct patterns of expression can identify chronic migraine from acute episodic migraine with some overlapping genes [46]. In this study, we identified both different activation of platelet genes and mitochondrial genes.

Further studies in chronic migraines have begun to elucidate patterns of response, contrasting patients that respond quickly to treatment versus patients that are slow to respond. These patterns of response may be due to alterations in calcium channel signaling, as well as neurotransmitter signaling in general. The identification of distinct patterns based on patients' responses appeared present prior to initial treatment and could separate this from medication-overuse headaches. Having these three distinct patterns of genomic expression (chronic migraine responders, medication-overuse headache responders versus nonresponders) and the potential predictability prior to treatment may further aid in not only the pathophysiological basis of migraine, chronic migraine and medication-overuse headaches, but also in identification of these patients at the onset of treatment to personalize their treatment methods.

7.1.4 Neuropeptides and transmitters

Several neuropeptides have been identified as having a role in pain modulation. These include the neurokinins (Substance P and Neurokinin A), the calcitonin gene-related peptide (CGRP) and vasoactive intestinal polypeptide (VIP). For migraine, CGRP appears to play an important role, with elevation in the headache phase of the migraine [47–49]. CGRP appears to act at the brainstem level and may be involved with the trigeminovascular complex. Owing to this observation, CGRP antagonists are in development and being tested for migraine treatment [50]. In addition, migraine prevention may be regulated by altering CGRP secretion and, thus, lower the potential for developing a migraine attack [51].

The predominant neurotransmitters that have been studied for migraine recently include serotonin and dopamine. Serotonin has been noted to have increased release from platelets during a migraine and may play an integral role in migraine propagation [52]. This led to the development of the triptans

(5-HT1B/D agonist) and their wide success in migraine treatment (Chapter 8). Dopamine has also been implicated in migraine pathophysiology, with many of the migraine features being able to be replicated by administering dopamine or dopamine agoinist [53]. This may also explain the effectiveness of dopamine antagonist for the acute treatment of migraine (Chapter 6) [54].

7.1.5 Factors influencing headache characteristics

As discussed in Chapters 2 and 3, primary headache disorders have defined characteristic features, some of which are used to define the diagnostic criteria (i.e. throbbing pain, associated features of nausea, vomiting, photophobia and phonophobia), while other features have begun to assist with both clinical characterization and with an understanding of the biological changes occurring in some migraineurs (i.e. cutaneous allodynia with central sensitization). An understanding of these clinical characteristics may help identify the pathphysiologic steps that are occurring during an individual attack.

Aura

The aura of a migraine is typically visual, sensory or dysphasic for migraine with aura by ICHD-II criteria with additional atypical aura including involvement of the motor systems (hemiplegic migraine) or brainstem (basilar-type migraine). The aura may be generated by a variety of pathophysiological changes, but the rate of spread of the typical aura has been correlated with the rate of the cortical spreading depression (CSD) of Leao [55]. CSD has been demonstrated in animals, and functional magnetic resonance imaging (fMRI) suggests that the same changes are occurring in humans that have migraine with aura [56]. The more complicated auras, however, may not be due to CSD, but have a genetic basis (as discussed above) as a channelopathy or energy production/deficit. The role of CSD and migraine has recently been reviewed and integrated into several of the molecular models [57].

Pain quality

Most migraineurs will describe the pain quality as a pulsatile or throbbing quality. Patients will frequently relate this feels like their heart beating in their head. Historically, this was one of the arguments of a vascular etiology to migraines. The vascular model proposes that, during a migraine attack, there is vascular dilation and plasma extravasations. The triggering mechanism for this vascular change is unclear, but it may represent increased cortical demands or a feedback loop from the trigeminal system. The dural vasculature is innervated by the first division of the trigeminal nerve. Several experimental models exist in an attempt to describe migraine pathophysiology and integrate the neurovascular basis with cranial vasodilation and trigeminal system activation [58].

This migraine-generated neurogenic edema and inflammation appears to be mediated via a trigeminovascular activation and feedback loop by the release of CGRP, Substance P and Neurokinin A. CGRP has been most strongly implicated [49], with its levels being altered during a migraine [59]. The activation of vasoactive peptides results in an inflammatory response within the blood vessels of the dura. This, alone, is not sufficient to cause a migraine, and there are likely central roles for CGRP [60]. CGRP has recently been shown to induce a migraine [61] and antagonism appears to abort a migraine [62], while current migraine agents block its release [51]. Nitric oxide has also been implicated to be involved in this vasoactive process [63–65]. This has been detected in the plasma of migraine and cluster headache patients and may represent a marker for migraine [66]. Alterations in transcription factors may also occur at the inception of migraine headache attacks, though their role remains very unclear [67].

Hypersensitivity

During a migraine attack, patients often complain of increased sensitivity to their surroundings. By diagnostic criteria, this includes sensitivity to light (photophobia) and sensitivity to sound (phonophobia). In addition, patients may complain of sensitivity to smells (osmophobia), as well as to the taste or texture of certain foods and to touch (cutaneous allodynia). This sensitivity may not only worsen during a headache, but be present at a lower level between attacks. One explanation for this observation is a lack of habituation to external stimuli. For auditory phenomena this is referred to as the passive 'oddball' auditory effect [69, 69]. In this procedure, nonmigraine subjects will attenuate to an auditory signal, while migraine patients have an increasing electrophysiological response.

One component of this heightened sensitivity that has recently been expanded on is cutaneous allodynia (a heightened skin sensitivity) with central sensitization [70, 71]. This observation was based on reports of scalp tenderness during migraine attacks [72–75], with the observation refined by the use of quantitative sensory testing (QST) [71]. Several modalities can be tested with QST, including thermal (heat and cold) and mechanical stimulation. Thermal testing has been standardized using the methods of limits [76, 77], while mechanical stimulation can be tested with either von Frey hairs (static or pressure allodynia) or gauze pads (dynamic or brush allodynia) [78]. The pressure allodynia has been standardized and demonstrated to be more sensitive [78].

With the use of QST the neuroanatomical pathways that are activated during an acute migraine are being identified [70], with evidence that a central activation of nociceptive neurons in the spinal trigeminal nucleus develops [79]. During a migraine attack, a patient's sensitivity to thermal or mechanical stimulation is increased. Initially, this appears to require ongoing activation of the central nuclei by the peripheral neurons (activity-dependent allodynia – early triptan administration), but with time the peripheral activation is no longer needed (activity-independent allodynia – late triptan administration). This observation has been demonstrated based on the response to treatment with triptans in humans with migraine [80] and in an animal inflammatory model using inflammatory soup applied to the dura (i.e. intracranial pain) and firing rates of individual neurons in the rat [81]. In a subset of patients with allodynia that becomes activity independent, it was found that COX1/COX2 inhibitors could reverse this activation, while another group of patients that had a history of opiod administration were unresponsive [82]. This suggests that there is a risk of disease progression that can be assessed in patients with allodynia based on their response pattern. This possible disease progression may represent a key point of intervention that can stop the progression of migraine. Thus, in children, we may be able to intervene early in the disease process and prevent long-term progression.

QST of all migraine patients is not feasible; thus, there has been a development of clinically viable tools for the assessment of allodynia in migraine patients, including clinical observations [83], questionnaires [84–87] and bedside testing [87, 88]. Although these methods have limitations compared with QST, combining these techniques with the patients' responses to treatment can improve the sensitivity up to 90% [86]. To date, the assessment of allodynia and validation of clinical-based questionnaires in children has not been reported. Given the phenotypical variability between patients and the potential progressive nature of migraine, the accurate identification of the development of both an activity-dependent and activity-independent allodynia should help better understand the evolution of migraine pathophysiology within patients and have a long-term impact on their outcome.

7.1.6 Neuroimaging

Neuroimaging studies, by positron emission tomography, single photon emission computed tomography (SPECT) and fMRI, have demonstrated changes in brain blood flow and metabolism change during acute migraine, with several changes localized to the brainstem [89–96].

SPECT can identify some of the changes in blood flow, which may be due to a spreading wave of depolarization accompanied by alterations in cerebral blood flow with both a transient decrease and increase (CSD) [57, 97]. As noted above, CSD may be responsible for the typical auras seen in migraine with aura. These alterations in blood flow have also been implicated in the etiology of the transient neurological changes that occur in these patients and appear to be suppressed by common therapeutic agents used in migraine prevention [98]. For migraine without aura, there have been no changes in regional blood flow, so CSD and blood flow changes appear to correlate only with the aura phase.

Neuroimaging studies, however, have begun to examine the potential of a migraine generator within the brainstem. Weiller *et al.* [90] first identified brainstem activation to be one of the initial steps in migraine initiation. This activation in patients with chronic migraine may lead to progressive changes in the brainstem in the periaqueductal gray matter [95]. Further refinement of neuroimagning techniques should help advance the understanding of the process involved in migraine and other primary headache propagation [94, 99].

7.2 TTHs: Tension-type headaches

Much less is known about the pathophysiology of TTHs. It has long been thought that there is a relationship to the pericranial muscles and subsequent increased activity resulting in the tightening feeling. This has historically led to the variety of names for TTH, including tension headache and muscle contraction headache.

One of the first questions to ask in the understanding of the mechanism of the TTH is whether it is an independent headache disorder or just a variant of migraine. Two models argue this point relating migraines and TTH. The continuum model suggests that migraine and TTH are a single pathophysiological disorder ranging from mild headaches (TTH) to moderate to severe headaches (migraine without aura) to the most severe headaches (migraines with aura) [100, 101]. This is in contrast to the spectrum model, which suggests that these are two separate entities, with the migraineurs having a full spectrum of headaches while the TTH patients have headaches limited to the mild to moderate pain disorder [102]. If the continuum model is correct, then focusing on the pathphysiology of migraine should help describe the mechanism of TTH, whereas TTH needs to be examined separately if the spectrum model is correct.

TTH may have a genetic basis, but this is much less clear than with migraine. Episodic TTH appears to be predominantly due to environmental changes [13], where the genetic basis of TTH appears to be more closely tied to chronic TTH [103, 104]. Ulrich *et al.* [13] examined the relative influence of genetic and environmental components for TTH in a twin-based study with 1417 subjects reporting TTH. In the general group they found the contribution of nonshared environmental factors was 81%, while the genetic factors had an additive contribution of 19%.

With the TTHs, there may be a secondary muscle contraction component, and some suggestion has been provided that this may enhance a feedback loop to build the TTH [105]. Recently, a role of central sensitization has been suggested and alternative theories have been reviewed [106, 107].

Other primary headaches

The other primary headaches occur with a very low frequency in children (Chapter 4) and with the exception of cluster headaches are also rare in adults. This has led to a limited understanding of the pathophysiology of these primary headache disorders, but there may be overlapping pathophysiology with migraine (reviewed by Edvinsson and Uddman [108]).

References

1. Prensky, A.L. and Sommer, D. (1979) Diagnosis and treatment of migraine in children. *Neurology*, **29**, 506–510.

2. Russell, M.B., Iselius, L. and Olesen, J. (1996) Migraine without aura and migraine with aura are inherited disorders. *Cephalalgia: An International Journal of Headache*, **16**, 305–309.

3. Russell, M.B. (1997) Genetic epidemiology of migraine and cluster headache. *Cephalalgia: An International Journal of Headache*, **17**, 683–701.

4. Kudrow, L. and Kudrow, D.B. (1994) Inheritance of cluster headache and its possible link to migraine. *Headache*, **34**(7), 400–407.

5. Ulrich, V., Gervil, M., Fenger, K. *et al.* (1999) The prevalence and characteristics of migraine in twins from the general population. *Headache*, **39**(3), 173–180.

6. Gervil, M., Ulrich, V., Kyvik, K.O. *et al.* (1999) Migraine without aura: a population-based twin study. *Annals of Neurology*, **46**(4), 606–611.

7. Svensson, D.A., Larsson, B., Bille, B. and Lichtenstein, P. (1999) Genetic and environmental influences on recurrent headaches in eight to nine-year-old twins. *Cephalalgia: An International Journal of Headache*, **19**(10), 866–872.

8. Kallela, M., Wessman, M. and Farkkila, M. (2001) Validation of a migraine-specific questionnaire for use in family studies. *European Journal of Neurology*, **8**(1), 61–66.

9. Kallela, M., Wessman, M., Havanka, H. *et al.* (2001) Familial migraine with and without aura: clinical characteristics and co-occurrence. *European Journal of Neurology*, **8**(5), 441–449.

10. Stewart, W.F., Bigal, M.E., Kolodner, K. *et al.* (2006) Familial risk of migraine: variation by proband age at onset and headache severity. *Neurology*, **66**(3), 344–348.

11. Gervil, M., Ulrich, V., Kaprio, J. *et al.* (1999) The relative role of genetic and environmental factors in migraine without aura. *Neurology*, **53**(5), 995–999.

12. Ulrich, V., Olesen, J., Gervil, M. and Russell, M.B. (2000) Possible risk factors and precipitants for migraine with aura in discordant twin-pairs: a population-based study. *Cephalalgia: An International Journal of Headache*, **20**(9), 821–825.

13. Ulrich, V., Gervil, M. and Olesen, J. (2004) The relative influence of environment and genes in episodic tension-type headache. *Neurology*, **62**(11), 2065–2069.

14. Peroutka, S.J., Price, S.C., Wilhoit, T.L. and Jones, K.W. (1998) Comorbid migraine with aura, anxiety, and depression is associated with dopamine D2 receptor (DRD2) *NcoI* alleles. *Molecular Medicine*, **4**, 14–21.

15. Montagna, P. (2000) Molecular genetics of migraine headaches: a review. *Cephalagia*, **20** 3–14.

16. Montagna, P. (2004) The physiopathology of migraine: the contribution of genetics. *Neurological Sciences*, **25** (Suppl 3), S93–S96.

17. Joutel, A., Bousser, M.G., Biousse, V. *et al.* (1993) A gene for familial hemiplegic migraine maps to chromosome 19. *Genetics*, **5**, 40–45.

18. Terwindt, G.M., Ophoff, R.A., Haan, J. *et al.* (1996) Familial hemiplegic migraine: a clinical comparison of families linked and unlinked to chromosome 19. *Cephalalgia: An International Journal of Headache*, **16**, 153–155.

19. Ophoff, R.A., Terwindt, G.M., Vergouwe, M.N. *et al.* (1996) Familial hemiplegic migraine and episodic ataxia type-2 are caused by mutations in the Ca^{2+} channel gene CACNL1A4. *Cell*, **87**, 544–552.

20. Terwindt, G.M., Ophoff, R.A., Haan, J. *et al.* (1998) Variable clinical expression of mutations in the P/Q-type calcium channel gene in familial hemiplegic migraine. *Neurology*, **50**, 1105–1110.

21. Carrera, P., Piatti, M., Stenirri, S. *et al.* (1999) Genetic heterogeneity in Italian families with familial hemiplegic migraine. *Neurology*, **53**(1), 26–33.

22. Gardner, K., Barmada, M., Ptacek, L.J. and Hoffman, E.P. (1997) A new locus for hemiplegic migraine maps to chromosome 1q31. *Neurology*, **49**, 1231–1238.

23. Marconi, R., De Fusco, M., Aridon, P. *et al.* (2003) Familial hemiplegic migraine type 2 is linked to 0.9Mb region on chromosome 1q23. *Annals of Neurology*, **53**(3), 376–381.

24. De Fusco, M., Marconi, R., Silvestri, L. *et al.* (2003) Haploinsufficiency of ATP1A2 encoding the Na^+/K^+ pump a2 subunit associated with familial hemiplegic migraine type 2. *Nature Genetics*, **33**(2), 192–196.

25. Moskowitz, M.A., Bolay, H. and Dalkara, T. (2004) Deciphering migraine mechanisms: clues from familial hemiplegic migraine genotypes. *Annals of Neurology*, **55**(2), 276–280.

26. Jurkat-Rott, K., Freilinger, T., Dreier, J.P. *et al.* (2004) Variability of familial hemiplegic migraine with novel A1A2 Na$^+$/K$^+$-ATPase variants. *Neurology*, **62**(10), 1857–1861.

27. Vanmolkot, K.R., Kors, E.E., Hottenga, J.J. *et al.* (2003) Novel mutations in the Na$^+$, K$^+$-ATPase pump gene ATP1A2 associated with familial hemiplegic migraine and benign familial infantile convulsions. *Annals of Neurology*, **54**(3), 360–366.

28. Swoboda, K.J., Kanavakis, E., Xaidara, A. *et al.* (2004) Alternating hemiplegia of childhood or familial hemiplegic migraine? A novel ATP1A2 mutation. *Annals of Neurology*, **55**(6), 884–887.

29. Dichgans, M., Freilinger, T., Eckstein, G. *et al.* (2005) Mutation in the neuronal voltage-gated sodium channel SCN1A in familial hemiplegic migraine. *Lancet*, **366**(9483), 371–377.

30. Ferrari, M.D. (1998) Migraine. *Lancet*, **351**, 1043–1051.

31. Welch, K.M.A. (1998) Current opinions in headache pathogenesis: introduction and synthesis. *Current Opinion in Neurology*, **11**, 193–197.

32. Cassidy, E.M., Tomkins, E., Dinan, T. *et al.* (2003) Central 5-HT receptor hypersensitivity in migraine without aura. *Cephalalgia: An International Journal of Headache*, **23**(1), 29–34.

33. Kaube, H., Katsarava, Z., Przywara, S. *et al.* (2002) Acute migraine headache: possible sensitization of neurons in the spinal trigeminal nucleus? *Neurology*, **58**(8), 1234–1238.

34. Katsarava, Z., Lehnerdt, G., Duda, B. *et al.* (2002) Sensitization of trigeminal nociception specific for migraine but not pain of sinusitis. *Neurology*, **59**(9), 1450–1453.

35. Siniatchkin, M., Kropp, P. and Gerber, W.D. (2003) What kind of habituation is impaired in migraine patients? *Cephalalgia: An International Journal of Headache*, **23**(7), 511–518.

36. De Marinis, M., Pujia, A., Natale, L. *et al.* (2003) Decreased habituation of the R2 component of the blink reflex in migraine patients. *Clinical Neurophysiology*, **114**(5), 889–893.

37. Katsarava, Z., Giffin, N., Diener, H.C. and Kaube, H. (2003) Abnormal habituation of 'nociceptive' blink reflex in migraine – evidence for increased excitability of trigeminal nociception. *Cephalalgia: An International Journal of Headache*, **23**(8), 814–819.

38. Bartsch, T., Knight, Y.E. and Goadsby, P.J. (2004) Activation of 5-HT(1B/1D) receptor in the periaqueductal gray inhibits nociception. *Annals of Neurology*, **56**(3), 371–381.

39. Kotani, K., Shimomura, T., Shimomura, F. *et al.* (2002) A polymorphism in the serotonin transporter gene regulatory region and frequency of migraine attacks. *Headache*, **42**(9), 893–895.

40. Borroni, B., Brambilla, C., Liberini, P. *et al.* (2005) Functional serotonin 5-HTTLPR polymorphism is a risk factor for migraine with aura. *The Journal of Headache and Pain*, **6**(4), 182–184.

41. Szilagyi, A., Boor, K., Orosz, I. *et al.* (2006) Contribution of serotonin transporter gene polymorphisms to pediatric migraine. *Headache*, **46**(3), 478–485.

42. Mossner, R., Weichselbaum, A., Marziniak, M. *et al.* (2005) A highly polymorphic poly-glutamine stretch in the potassium channel KCNN3 in migraine. *Headache*, **45**(2), 132–136.

43. Scher, A.I., Terwindt, G.M., Verschuren, W.M. *et al.* (2006) Migraine and MTHFR C677T genotype in a population-based sample. *Annals of Neurology*, **59**(2), 372–375.

44. Schürks, M., Kurth, T., Geissler, I. *et al.* (2006) Cluster headache is associated with the G1246A polymorphism in the hypocretin receptor 2 gene. *Neurology*, **66**(12), 1917–1919.

45. Baumber, L., Sjostrand, C., Leone, M. *et al.* (2006) A genome-wide scan and HCRTR2 candidate gene analysis in a European cluster headache cohort. *Neurology*, **66**(12), 1888–1893.

46. Tang, Y., Hershey, A.D., Powers, S.W. *et al.* (2004) Genomic abnormalities in patients with migraine and chronic migraine: preliminary blood gene expression suggests platelet abnormalities. *Headache*, **44**(10), 994–1004.

47. Goadsby, P.J., Edvinsson, L. and Ekman, R. (1990) Vasoactive peptide release in the extracerebral circulation of humans during migraine headache. *Annals of Neurology*, **28**, 183–187.

48. Gallai, V., Sarchielli, P., Floridi, A. *et al.* (1995) Vasoactive peptide levels in the plasma of young migraine patients with and without aura assessed both interictally and ictally. *Cephalalgia: An International Journal of Headache*, **15**(5), 384–390.

49. Durham, P.L. (2006) Calcitonin gene-related peptide (CGRP) and migraine. *Headache*, **46** (Suppl 1), S3–S8.

50. Doods, H., Arndt, K., Rudolf, K. and Just, S. (2007) CGRP antagonists: unravelling the role of CGRP in migraine. *Trends in Pharmacological Sciences*, **28**(11), 580–587.

51. Durham, P.L., Niemann, C. and Cady, R. (2006) Repression of stimulated calcitonin gene-related peptide secretion by topiramate. *Headache*, **46**(8), 1291–1295.

52. Hamon, M. and Bourgoin, S. (2000) Role of serotonin and other neuroactive molecules in the physiopathogenesis of migraine. Current hypotheses. *Pathologie–Biologie*, **48**(7), 619–629.

53. Peroutka, S.J. (1997) Dopamine and migraine. *Neurology*, **49**, 650–656.

54. Akerman, S. and Goadsby, P.J. (2007) Dopamine and migraine: biology and clinical implications. *Cephalalgia: An International Journal of Headache*, **27**(11), 1308–1314.

55. Lauritzen, M. (1994) Pathophysiology of the migraine aura. The spreading depression theory. *Brain: A Journal of Neurology*, **117** (Pt 1), 199–210.

56. Hadjikhani, N., Sanchez Del Rio, M., Wu, O. *et al.* (2001) Mechanisms of migraine aura revealed by functional MRI in human visual cortex. *Proceedings of the National Academy of Sciences of the United States of America* **98**(8), 4687–4692.

57. Moskowitz, M.A. (2007) Pathophysiology of headache – past and present. *Headache*, **47** (Suppl 1), S58–S63.

58. Arulmani, U., Gupta, S., VanDenBrink, A.M. *et al.* (2006) Experimental migraine models and their relevance in migraine therapy. *Cephalalgia: An International Journal of Headache*, **26**(6), 642–659.

59. Bellamy, J.L., Cady, R.K. and Durham, P.L. (2006) Salivary levels of CGRP and VIP in rhinosinusitis and migraine patients. *Headache*, **46**(1), 24–33.

60. Levy, D., Burstein, R. and Strassman, A.M. (2005) Calcitonin gene-related peptide does not excite or sensitize meningeal nociceptors: implications for the pathophysiology of migraine. *Annals of Neurology*, **58**(5), 698–705.

61. Lassen, L.H., Haderslev, P.A., Jacobsen, V.B. *et al.* (2002) CGRP may play a causative role in migraine. *Cephalalgia: An International Journal of Headache*, **22**, 54–61.

62. Edvinsson, L. (2005) Clinical data on the CGRP antagonist BIBN4096BS for treatment of migraine attacks. *CNS Drug Reviews*, **11**(1), 69–76.

63. Griffiths, L.R., Nyholt, D.R., Curtain, R.P. *et al.* (1997) Migraine association and linkage studies of an endothelial nitric oxide synthase (NOS3) gene polymorphism. *Neurology*, **49**, 614–617.

64. Olesen, J., Thomsen, L.L., Lassen, L.H. and Olesen, I.J. (1995) The nitric oxide hypothesis of migraine and other vascular headaches. *Cephalalgia: An International Journal of Headache*, **15**, 94–100.

65. Thomsen, L.L. and Olesen, J. (1998) Nitric oxide theory of migraine. *Clinical Neuroscience (New York, NY)*, **5**, 28–33.

66. D'Amico, D., Ferraris, A., Leone, M. *et al.* (2002) Increased plasma nitrates in migraine and cluster headache patients in interictal periods: basal hyperactivity of L-argingine-NO pathway? *Cephalalgia: An International Journal of Headache*, **22**, 33–36.

67. Reutter, U., Chiarugi, A., Bolay, H. and Moskowitz, M.A. (2002) Nuclear factor-KB as a molecular target for migraine therapy. *Annals of Neurology*, **51**, 507–516.

68. Schoenen, J. (1998) Cortical electrophysiology in migraine and possible pathogenetic implications. *Clinical Neuroscience (New York, NY)*, **5**(1), 10–17.

69. Wang, W. and Schoenen, J. (1998) Interictal potentiation of passive 'oddball' auditory event-related potentials in migraine. *Cephalalgia: An International Journal of Headache*, **18**(5), 261–265; discussion, 41.

70. Burstein, R., Cutrer, M.F. and Yarnitsky, D. (2000) The development of cutaneous allodynia during a migraine attack clinical evidence for the sequential recruitment of spinal and supraspinal nociceptive neurons in migraine. *Brain: A Journal of Neurology*, **123**(Pt 8), 1703–1709.

71. Burstein, R., Yarnitsky, D., Goor-Aryeh, I. *et al.* (2000) An association between migraine and cutaneous allodynia. *Annals of Neurology*, **47**(5), 614–624.

72. Drummond, P.D. (1987) Scalp tenderness and sensitivity to pain in migraine and tension headache. *Headache*, **27**(1), 45–50.

73. Jensen, K., Tuxen, C. and Olesen, J. (1988) Pericranial muscle tenderness and pressure-pain threshold in the temporal region during common migraine. *Pain*, **35**(1), 65–70.

74. Jensen, R., Rasmussen, B.K., Pedersen, B. and Olesen, J. (1993) Muscle tenderness and pressure pain thresholds in headache. A population study. *Pain*, **52**(2), 193–199.

75. Lous, I. and Olesen, J. (1982) Evaluation of pericranial tenderness and oral function in patients with common migraine, muscle contraction headache and 'combination headache'. *Pain*, **12**(4), 385–393.

76. Fruhstorfer, H., Lindblom, U. and Schmidt, W.C. (1976) Method for quantitative estimation of thermal thresholds in patients. *Journal of Neurology, Neurosurgery, and Psychiatry*, **39**(11), 1071–1075.

77. Yarnitsky, D. (1997) Quantitative sensory testing. *Muscle & Nerve*, **20**(2), 198–204.

78. LoPinto, C., Young, W.B. and Ashkenazi, A. (2006) Comparison of dynamic (brush) and static (pressure) mechanical allodynia in migraine. *Cephalalgia: An International Journal of Headache*, **26**(7), 852–856.

79. Yarnitsky, D., Goor-Aryeh, I., Bajwa, Z.H. *et al.* (2003) Wolff Award: possible parasympathetic contributions to peripheral and central sensitization during migraine. *Headache*, **43**(7), 704–714.

80. Burstein, R., Collins, B. and Jakubowski, M. (2004) Defeating migraine pain with triptans: a race against the development of cutaneous allodynia. *Annals of Neurology*, **55**(1), 19–26.

81. Burstein, R. and Jakubowski, M. (2004) Analgesic triptan action in an animal model of intracranial pain: a race against the development of central sensitization. *Annals of Neurology*, **55**(1), 27–36.

82. Jakubowski, M., Levy, D., Goor-Aryeh, I. *et al.* (2005) Terminating migraine with allodynia and ongoing central sensitization using parenteral administration of COX1/ COX2 inhibitors. *Headache*, **45**(7), 850–861.

83. Mathew, N.T., Kailasam, J. and Seifert, T. (2004) Clinical recognition of allodynia in migraine. *Neurology*, **63**(5), 848–852.

84. Jakubowski, M., Silberstein, S., Ashkenazi, A. and Burstein, R. (2005) Can allodynic migraine patients be identified interictally using a questionnaire? *Neurology*, **65**(9), 1419–1422.

85. Landy, S.H., McGinnis, J.E. and McDonald, S.A. (2007) Clarification of developing and established clinical allodynia and pain-free outcomes. *Headache*, **47**(2), 247–252.

86. Ashkenazi, A., Silberstein, S., Jakubowski, M. and Burstein, R. (2007) Improved identification of allodynic migraine patients using a questionnaire. *Cephalalgia: An International Journal of Headache*, **27**(4), 325–329.

87. Young, W.B., Richardson, E.S. and Shukla, P. (2005) Brush allodynia in hospitalized headache patients. *Headache*, **45**(8), 999–1003.

88. Ashkenazi, A., Sholtzow, M., Shaw, J.W. *et al.* (2007) Identifying cutaneous allodynia in chronic migraine using a practical clinical method. *Cephalalgia: An International Journal of Headache*, **27**(2), 111–117.

89. Sanchez del Rio, M., Bakker, D., Wu, O. *et al.* (1999) Perfusion weighted imaging during migraine: spontaneous visual aura and headache. *Cephalalgia: An International Journal of Headache*, **19**, 701–707.

90. Weiller, C., May, A., Limmroth, V. *et al.* (1995) Brain stem activation in spontaneous human migraine attacks. *Nature Medicine*, **1**(7), 658–660.

91. Woods, R.P., Iacoboni, M. and Mazziotta, J.C. (1994) Bilateral spreading of cerebral hypoperfusion during spontaneous migraine headache. *The New England Journal of Medicine*, **331**, 1689–1692.

92. Goadsby, P.J. (2005) Migraine pathophysiology. *Headache*, **45** (Suppl 1), S14–S24.

93. Goadsby, P.J. (2001) Neuroimaging in headache. *Microscopy Research and Technique*, **53**(3), 179–187.

94. Cohen, A.S. and Goadsby, P.J. (2006) Functional neuroimaging of primary headache disorders. *Expert Review of Neurotherapeutics*, **6**(8), 1159–1171.

95. Welch, K.M., Nagesh, V., Aurora, S.K. and Gelman, N. (2001) Periaqueductal gray matter dysfunction in migraine: cause or the burden of illness? *Headache*, **41**(7), 629–637.

96. Borsook, D., Burstein, R., Moulton, E. and Becerra, L. (2006) Functional imaging of the trigeminal system: applications to migraine pathophysiology. *Headache*, **46** (Suppl 1), S32–S38.

97. Choudhuri, R., Cui, L., Yong, C. *et al.* (2002) Cortical spreading depression and gene regulation: relevance to migraine. *Annals of Neurology*, **51**(4), 499–506.

98. Ayata, C., Jin, H., Kudo, C. *et al.* (2006) Suppression of cortical spreading depression in migraine prophylaxis. *Annals of Neurology*, **59**(4), 652–661.

99. DaSilva, A.F., Goadsby, P.J. and Borsook, D., (2007) Cluster headache: a review of neuroimaging findings. *Current Pain and Headache Reports*, **11**(2), 131–136.

100. Viswanathan, V., Bridges, S.J., Whitehouse, W. and Newton, R.W. (1998) Childhood headaches: discrete entities or continuum? *Developmental Medicine and Child Neurology*, **40**(8), 544–550.

101. Cady, R., Schreiber, C., Farmer, K. and Sheftell, F. (2002) Primary headaches: A convergence hypothesis. *Headache*, **42**, 204–216.

102. Lipton, R.B., Stewart, W.F., Cady, R. *et al.* (2000) Sumatriptan for the range of headaches in migraine sufferers: results of the Spectrum Study. *Headache*, **40**, 783–791.

103. Ostergaard, S., Russell, M.B., Bendtsen, L. and Olesen, J. (1997) Comparison of first degree relatives and spouses of people with chronic tension headache. *BMJ (Clinical Research)*, **314**(7087), 1092–1093.

104. Russell, M.B., Ostergaard, S., Bendtsen, L. and Olesen, J. (1999) Familial occurrence of chronic tension-type headache. *Cephalalgia: An International Journal of Headache*, **19**(4), 207–210.

105. Langemark, M. and Olesen, J. (1987) Pericranial tenderness in tension headache. A blind, controlled study. *Cephalalgia: An International Journal of Headache*, **7**(4), 249–255.

106. Jensen, R. (1999) Pathophysiological mechanisms of tension-type headache: a review of epidemiological and experimental studies. *Cephalalgia: An International Journal of Headache*, **19**(6), 602–621.

107. Bendtsen, L. (2000) Central sensitization in tension-type headache – possible pathophysiological mechanisms. *Cephalalgia: An International Journal of Headache*, **20**(5), 486–508.

108. Edvinsson, L. and Uddman, R. (2005) Neurobiology in primary headaches. *Brain Research*, **48**(3), 438–456.

8
Migraine: diagnosis and treatment

Paul Winner

Migraine in the pediatric population is frequently not recognized and remains underdiagnosed and undertreated. This may be due to both the patient's and parent's impression of what a migraine is and the clinician's reliance on experience rather than standardized diagnosis. Standardized criteria have been developed that address this problem and have recently been revised. The International Classification of Headache Disorders (ICHD-II) is an improvement and should assist with the proper diagnosis.

Once the correct diagnosis is established, a treatment plan can be developed. This often entails a combination of acute and preventative therapies and biobehavioral interventions. Goals of treatment should be clearly established for the patients and parents, and realistic time courses discussed.

8.1 Diagnosis

The high prevalence of migraine in children and adolescents makes it essential that an accurate diagnosis be made. The most resent criteria, ICHD-II, represents an improvement in the standardized criteria, though it was developed primarily for headache disorders in adults [1]. ICHD-II is based on the 1988 ICHD-I [2], which has been revised after clinical use, though it remained a work in progress. Several studies on the diagnosis of pediatric headache have provided a basis for the recommended revisions to the ICHD-II criteria for

Pediatric Headaches in Clinical Practice   Andrew D. Hershey, Paul Winner, Marielle A. Kabbouche and Scott W. Powers
© 2009 John Wiley & Sons, Ltd.

pediatric migraine [3–8]. Continued revisions and emerging new criteria should provide important tools for clinical practice, clinical trials and epidemiologic research.

Headaches can be divided into primary headaches (i.e. those intrinsic to the nervous system) and secondary headaches (i.e. those directly attributed to another cause). In the ICHD-II system, the primary headache disorders (migraine, tension-type headache and cluster headache) are defined based on the symptom profiles and on the pattern of headache attacks. The general medical and neurologic examinations, as well as diagnostic tests, serve primarily to exclude secondary headaches. In the absence of a diagnostic gold standard or specific biomarkers, clinicians and researchers have struggled to develop valid and reliable diagnostic criteria for specific headache subtypes and phenotypic variations.

Migraine and tension-type headache are the most frequently seen recurrent, episodic headaches in childhood. Although the ICHD-II criteria view migraine and tension-type headache as distinct disorders, they are sometimes regarded as a continuum based on severity [9–11]. Other views, however, suggest that they are distinct disorders, with migraine having a spectrum of symptoms and severity in different attacks [12].

Part of this confusion is due to the recognition that migraine is a heterogeneous disorder that can vary between attacks in pain intensity, duration, pattern of associated features and frequency of occurrence [13]. This lack of consistency in disease manifestations among children complicates the establishment of highly sensitive and specific criteria. In the pediatric population this may be further complicated to the evolution of symptoms over time, either due to a change in the phenotype or due to the child's ability to describe the symptoms. In addition, the effects of treatment, both acute and preventative, can modify the presentation of the disease. This can lead to both exacerbations and remissions in children. Because both clinicians and epidemiologists must rely on the recall of patients or parents, diagnoses are subject to recall bias.

Pediatric migraine diagnostic criteria

Vahlquist and Hackzell, followed by Bille, defined migraine as paroxysmal headaches separated by symptom-free intervals and accompanied by at least two of four features: (1) unilaterality, (2) nausea, (3) visual aura and (4) family history of migraine [14, 15]. In 1962, the Ad Hoc Committee on Classification of Headaches provided a description of migraine, but did not specify which features had to be present to make a diagnosis [16].

In 1988, the International Headache Society (IHS) proposed a set of criteria for migraine headaches based on international expert consensus [2]. These criteria had few allowances for the diagnosis of pediatric headaches and they have been challenged primarily due to disagreement between expert clinical diagnosis and IHS-based diagnosis, with reported levels of agreement ranging from 44 to 66% [3–5, 7, 17–20]. The sensitivity of the IHS criteria suggests that these criteria are more restrictive in comparison with expert clinical diagnosis. This may be problematic in clinical practice, where a clinician usually assigns a diagnosis as a prelude to treatment.

Young children and their parents may not be able to describe the pain or the associated features of the attacks in the terms required by the IHS criteria, while in some instances vomiting and abdominal discomfort may overshadow the complaint of headache. In their specialty center-based study, Seshia et al. [7] found that, in children with headaches, 30% could not describe the quality of their pain and 16% could not report on photophobia and phonophobia.

The criticisms of the HIS criteria have resulted in some of the changes noted in the ICHD-II criteria as they relate to this patient population [1] (Table 8.1). The ICHD-II criteria recognizes shorter headache duration for patients (1 to 72 h). Of those with a clinical diagnosis of migraine, 11–81% have a headache duration of less than 2 h and 8–25% have a headache duration of less than 1 h. Several investigators, therefore, have argued that the minimum duration required for diagnosis should be reduced from 2 h to 1 h. Winner et al. [18] reported that making this reduction increased the diagnostic sensitivity from 66% to 78% using clinical diagnosis as the gold standard. Maytal et al. [5] showed that decreasing the minimal duration to less than 1 h produced small gains in the sensitivity but substantially reduced the specificity of the definition in one study.

The validity of the ICHD-II criteria continues to be tested in the pediatric population [21, 22]. In comparing ICHD-I (IHS criteria) with ICHD-II, with the clinical impression serving as the gold standard, Lima et al. [21] found that the sensitivity for the diagnosis of migraine without aura increased from 21% to 53%, while for migraine with aura it increased from 27% to 71%. There was no change in the specificity of the criteria. In a study by the American Headache Society Pediatric–Adolescent Section, this change was not as dramatic; but it was found that, if short-duration headaches were allowed, the ICHD-II criteria diagnosed 80.8% [22]. Further modifications suggested by this analysis included allowing for focal location, and short duration increased this sensitivity further to 84.4%.

Table 8.1   ICHD-II criteria for migraine without aura. (ICHD-II criteria reproduced with permission from Blackwell Publishing)

Previously used terms
Common migraine, hemicrania simplex

Description
Recurrent headache disorder manifesting in attacks lasting 4–72 h. Typical characteristics of the headache are unilateral location, pulsation quality, moderate or severe intensity, aggravation by routine physical activity and association with nausea and/or photophobia and phonophobia.

Diagnostic criteria
A.   At least five attacks fulfilling criteria B–D
B.   Headache attacks lasting 4–72 h (untreated or unsuccessfully treated) [2–4]
C.   Headache has at least two of the following characteristics:
    1.   unilateral location [5, 6]
    2.   pulsating quality [7]
    3.   moderate or severe pain intensity
    4.   aggravation by or causing avoidance of routine physical activity (e.g. walking or climbing stairs)
D.   During headache at least one of the following:
    1.   nausea and/or vomiting
    2.   photophobia and phonophobia [8]
E.   Not attributed to another disorder [9]

Notes
1.   Differentiating between 1.1 *Migraine without aura* and 2.1 *Infrequent episodic tension-type headache* may be difficult. Therefore, at least five attacks are required. Individuals who otherwise meet criteria for 1.1 *Migraine without aura* but have had fewer than five attacks should be coded 1.6.1 *Probable migraine without aura.*
2.   When the patient falls asleep during migraine and wakes up without it, duration of the attack is reckoned until the time of awakening.
3.   In children, attacks may last 1–72 h (although the evidence for the untreated durations of less than 2 h in children requires corroboration by prospective diary studies).
4.   When attacks occur on ≥15 days per month for >3 months, code as 1.1 *Migraine without aura* and as 1.5.1 *Chronic migraine.*
5.   Migraine headache is commonly bilateral in young children; an adult pattern of unilateral pain usually emerges in late adolescent or early adult life.
6.   Migraine headache is usually frontotemporal. Occipital headache in *children,* whether unilateral or bilateral, is rare and calls for diagnostic caution; many cases are attributable to structural lesions.
7.   *Pulsating* means throbbing or varying with the heartbeat.
8.   In young children, photophobia and phonophobia may be inferred from their behavior.
9.   History and physical and neurological examinations do not suggest any of the disorders listed in groups 5–12, or history and/or physical and/or neurological examinations do not suggest such disorder but it is ruled out by appropriate investigations, or such disorder is present but attacks do not occur for the first time in close temporal relation to the disorder [1].

Unilateral pain has been challenged as a diagnostic criterion because it is more characteristic of adult migraine than of pediatric migraine. Metsahonkala and Sillanpaa reported that 67% of their migraineurs had unilateral pain, while Gallai *et al.* found that 41.5% of their IHS migraineurs had unilateral pain and Maytal *et al.* found that unilateral pain had a sensitivity of 34% and a specificity of 86% using clinical diagnosis as the gold standard [3, 5, 20, 23]. The ICHD–II criteria note that migraine is commonly bilateral in young children; an adult pattern of unilateral pain usually emerges in late adolescence or early adult life. It has also been noted that migraine is usually frontatemporal. Occipital headache in children, whether unilateral or bilateral, is rare and calls for diagnostic caution, as many cases maybe attributable to structural lesions.

Several factors may account for the difficulty in improving agreement between clinical and criteria-based diagnosis of pediatric migraine. Diagnosticians may rely on features of migraine that are not included in the current diagnostic criteria. Some children with migraine have atypical presentations, including recurrent episodes of abdominal pain or vertigo with or without headache. In addition, young children may not be able to describe the pain or the associated features of the attacks in the terms required by the ICHD-II criteria.

The history is central in determining the correct diagnosis; the questions need to be directed to both the child and the parents. Children can provide useful information if questions are phrased in their language. A separate interview with the adolescent patient is recommended. Use of questionnaires and a structured interview format that is developmentally appropriate can assist with this evaluation. A detailed description of this evaluation can be found elsewhere and guidelines have been established regarding further testing [24, 25].

The headache history needs to include a detailed description of the headache episode, including any premonitory symptoms and triggers. The presence of an aura needs to be addressed and may be an unusual concept for young children to understand. Specific headache characteristics to address include cranial location of the pain, severity and quality of the pain, associated symptoms, alteration in activity level, frequency and duration of attacks, impact of the disease in terms of disability and quality of life. The frequency needs to address the number of headaches, as well as the number of days per month. Disability can be assessed using standardized tools that are widely available [23, 26, 27].

The medical history in the pediatric population should include details concerning pregnancy, labor and delivery, growth and development, previous injuries (especially head injuries), operations, hospitalizations, serious illnesses, drug allergies, current medications, use of illicit drugs or alcohol. A review of systems is necessary to establish whether there may be other causes of headache that will need to be addressed. A family history of headache should be obtained; additional history of hypertension, allergy, collagen vascular disease, epilepsy, tumor and neurocutaneous disorders is recommended.

There should be a comprehensive physical examination, including a detailed neurological and comprehensive headache examination, which should be preformed with special attention to gait abnormalities, since posterior fossa lesions will cause a wide-based, unsteady gait [28]. The head circumference should be measured in young children. If significantly enlarged, then familial macrocephaly, hydrocephalus and neurofibromatosis are in the differential. The presence of a cranial bruit may indicate an underlying vascular abnormality. In young children, the funduscopic examination is best performed at the end of the examination. In the majority of patients with migraine headaches, the general physical and neurologic examinations are normal.

Further testing is usually not warranted unless secondary headaches are suspected; for example, if there are abnormalities in the neurological examination, the headaches are primarily occipital in location or there are acute changes in the headache features [24]. In these cases, magnetic resonance imaging is recommended to exclude any intracranial pathology.

8.2 Treatment

The treatment of primary headache disorders in children includes acute therapy, preventative therapy and biobehavioral therapy. The meta-analysis of the pharmacologic treatment of childhood headaches has been completed, as well as a practice parameter developed and reviewed [29].

Acute therapy will need to be outlined for all children. The treatment is designed to stop episodic headaches. The goal of this treatment should be a quick response with return to normal activity and without relapse. A typical time course is resolution and return to normal functioning within 1 to 2 h. The second component of treatment is preventative treatment, which will need to be considered on a case-by-case basis. When a child's headaches are frequent (more than three or four headaches per month) or there is significant disability based on standardized assessment tools such as PedMIDAS, preventative treatment should be considered with a goal of minimizing the impact of the headache while reducing the number [23, 30]. This may not result in complete resolution, but an improvement to one or two headaches per month with minimal impact. The final component of treatment is biobehavioral therapy. This is a complex treatment that involves normalizing a child's lifestyle, as well as establishing long-term health goals and promoting proper medication use.

Acute treatment

Presently there are no Food and Drug Administration (FDA)-approved medications for the treatment of migraine in the prediatric population. Primarily, over-the-counter medications are often utilized, including non-steroidal anti-inflammatory drugs (NSAIDs: ibuprofen, naproxen sodium, and for older children aspirin) and general pain relievers (acetaminophen). Most prescriptive nonspecific medications have either not been evaluated in children or have not been proven statistically effective. Many prescriptive medications contain sedatives or narcotics that may treat the pain, but do not allow the child to return to normal functioning. Migraine-specific medications, including the triptans and dihydroergotamine (DHE), have been approved for adult use but remain under evaluation in the pediatric population. These medications have been demonstrated to be effective in more recent studies; however, they are yet to be approved by the FDA for use in children and adolescents.

For the nonspecific medications, Hämäläinen et al. [31] reported a comparative, double-blinded, placebo-controlled, crossover study of placebo versus ibuprofen versus acetaminophen. Eighty-eight children with a clear diagnosis of migraine participated. These patients treated a migraine headache with placebo, ibuprofen at a dose of 10 mg/kg or acetaminophen at a dose of 15 mg/kg. Improvement in headache relief and pain freedom were assessed. The results of this study indicated that ibuprofen was superior to both placebo and acetaminophen at both the 1 and 2 h time points, while acetaminophen did become superior to placebo at 2 h. Lewis et al. [32] performed a similar study on a group of younger children using a dose of ibuprofen at 7.5 mg/kg versus placebo with a similar outcome, although there was a slight male-to-female difference.

Based on these studies and the tolerability of ibuprofen, it has become a mainstay for the acute treatment of childhood headache and migraines. Proper use of ibuprofen requires the child to learn to identify the onset of the headache in order to initiate rapid treatment, use the proper dose based on their weight and avoid overuse, typically limiting it to not more than two to three times per week.

When NSAIDs are ineffective or partially effective, migraine-specific therapy is often required. Triptans are 5HT-1$_{B/D}$ agonists, migraine-specific medications. There are currently seven triptans approved for use in the USA in adults, but none is approved for the use of childhood or adolescent migraine. Several studies have demonstrated their effectiveness, including the use of sumatriptan both in tablet and nasal spray formulatons.

One of the initial studies in children was subcutaneous sumatriptan at a 0.06 mg/kg dose. The overall effectiveness was 72% at 30 min, and 78% at 2 h, with a low recurrence rate of 6% [33]. Injection of medication is often rejected by children, and this has limited its use.

Oral sumatriptan has been studied in a double-blinded, placebo control study with 25, 50 and 100 mg tablets [34]. The study's primary endpoint was at 2 h headache response and statistical significance was not reached due to a high placebo rate. Sumatriptan was statistically significant over the placebo at 25, 50 and 100 mg at both the 3 and 4 mark, with 74% pain relief at the 4 h mark. Headache recurrence rate remained lower in children than adults at 18–28% for sumatriptan, with no significant adverse affects seen.

Sumatriptan nasal spray has been studied in a randomized double-blinded placebo control trial in adolescents from 12 to 17 years, for a single attack, using 5, 10 and 20 mg doses [35]. At 1 h, 56% of patients using the 20 mg dose reported significant headache relief, compared with 41% with placebo. If pain-free response is examined, then the 20 mg dose was statistically significant with a 46% response rate at 2 h, compared with 25% for placebo. Associated symptoms were lower in the active medication group, with photophobia significantly lower with the 20 mg dose in 2 h. An additional nasal sumatriptan study using 5 mg, 20 mg and placebo dosing in a one-to-one ratio with 738 adolescents did demonstrate that, at 30 min, a 20 mg dose had a greater headache relief (42% versus 33%, $p = 0.046$) [36]. At 1 h, this increased to 61% for active medicine versus 52% placebo (not significant). By 2 h, response was increased to 68% for sumatriptan versus 58% for placebo ($p = 0.025$). There was also increased sustained release 1 through 24 h and 2 through 24 h.

Additonally, rizatriptan 5 mg tablets have also been evaluated in the 12–17 years age group, with a double-blinded placebo-controlled parallel group single attack study [37]. Of 149 adolescents using rizatriptan compared with 147 using placebo, the response rate at 2 h for the rizatriptan group was 66%, whereas the placebo affect was 57%. The response of 66% in this study was comparable to the adult studies, but the placebo dose was much greater than reported in adults. Headache-free rate at 2 h was 32% for the rizatriptan group, compared with 28% in the placebo group, with no serious adverse effects noted.

Zolmitriptan has also been studied in adolescents at both the 2.5 mg and 5 mg doses [38]. The response rate was 88% and 70% respectively, with the treatment well tolerated. Nasal zolmitriptan was recently found to be effective using a unique study design to minimize the placebo response rate. Two hundred and forty-eight adolescents were studied in a randomized, double-blind, placebo-controlled, two-attack crossover trial with a single-blind placebo challenge. Seventy-seven patients responded to the placebo challenge and did not continue in the analysis. In the remaining 171 patients, zolmitriptan produced significantly higher headache response rates than placebo at 1 h post-dose (58.1% versus 43.3%; $p < 0.02$), with an onset of action as early as 15 min. Zolmitriptan also produced significant pain-free response at 1 h (27.7% versus placebo 10.2%, $p < 0.001$) and the adolescents experienced a lower incidence of adverse events than usually seen in adults, with no serious adverse events or withdrawals.

Two methods may be utilized for triptan use [39]. One is the rescue therapy, where the child starts with an NSAID at an appropriate dose at the onset of their headaches. If they recognize that this is not working, then a triptan is used as rescue therapy. The alternative method requires the patient to determine the headache severity at the onset. They take their NSAIDs for a mild or moderate headache, whereas they take their triptans for moderate to severe headaches. This, however, has not been successful in children, as they oftentimes have difficulty recognizing the headache severity at its onset. In addition, combined therapy may be even more effective due to the multimechanism model of treatment [40].

Reports have shown the usefulness of intravenous DHE in an inpatient setting to break status migrainosus or prolonged migraines in children, and may have further benefit if premedicated with dopamine antagonists such as promethazine hydrochloride or metoclopramide hydrochloride [41]. More recently, nasal DHE has been used in adults. The extrapolation of the use in children and adolescents remains limited.

Dopamine antagonists, including prochlorperazine and metoclopramide, were initially used to control the nausea and vomiting effects of migraine [42]. Subsequently, the dopaminergic model of migraine was developed, and these compounds have been reanalyzed for usefulness in acute therapy [43]. The current uses need to be cautioned due to the development of extrapyramidal side effects. An open labeled study in 20 children did demonstrate the effectiveness of prochlorperazine in the emergency room setting [44]. These can often be used to break an acute episode of status migrainosus.

Burstein *et al.* [45] have identified cutaneous allodynia with central sensitization in adult migraine patients. In patients that do get allodynia with central sensitization, there is a reported decreased response to medication once the allodynia has been established [46, 47]. If a patient is identified as having allodynia, then it becomes important to stress the need for early treatment.

It is important to review the proper use of acute medications in order to avoid the potential for medication overuse. Acute medication should not roughly exceed two to three days per week. Medication overuse or analgesic rebound headaches are felt to be a frequent cause of transformed migraines or chronic daily headaches.

Prophylactic medication

Preventative therapy needs to be considered when headache or migraine becomes highly frequent or disabling. The goal of preventative treatment is reduction of headache frequency, as well as improvement of headache disability. In addition, a clear diminishment in severity and associated features may also be observed. Presently, there has not been a single preventative medication approved for the treatment of childhood migraine. Several studies have demonstrated the effectiveness of some of these medications. Preventative medication is largely grouped into antiepileptic medications, antidepressant medications, antiserotonergic medications, and antihypertensive medications.

The antiepileptic medications currently being used for the prevention of migraine include divalproate sodium, topiramate, gabapentin, levetiracetam and zonisamide. Currently, for the prevention of adult migraines, both divalproate sodium and topiramate are approved by the FDA [48, 49]. The effective dose in the pediatric population for both of these medications is not known, but a dose of approximately 15–20 mg/kg per day for divalproate sodium and a dose of 2–4 mg/kg per day for topiramate appear to be effective. To achieve this dose, however, it must be tapered slowly, typically increasing the dose in quarter steps over 8–12 weeks. For divalproate, a study of 31 children aged 7–16 years showed at a dose of 15–45 mg/kg a 76% responsiveness of a greater than 50% reduction in their headache frequency, while 18% had a greater than 75% reduction and 6% were headache free [50]. A study using standardized doses of either 500 or 1000 mg of divalproate in 9–17-year-olds also reported a reduction in severity of the visual analog scale from 6.8 to 0.7, with a decrease in headache frequency from 6 per month to 0.7 per month [51].

In an open label study, topiramate did demonstrate its effectiveness [52]. In a study of 162 children from age 6 to 15 years, using a dose of 2–3 mg/kg per day, with a maximum dose of topiramate 200 mg, resulted in a reduced mean frequency of migraine from 5.4 days per month to 1.9 days per month [53]. Although not statistically significant, it did trend that way ($p = 0.065$); this was felt to be due to a large variation in the placebo-response group.

Amitriptyline has been used for many decades for its antidepressive properties, and was first recognized in the 1970s as an effective migraine therapy in adults [54–56]. Most of the studies in children with amitriptyline have been open label studies with no placebo-controlled studies. Levinstein [57], comparing amitriptyline with propranolol and cyproheptadine, found amitriptyline to be effective in 50–60% of the children. In an open label pediatric study, amitriptyline resulted in a perceived improvement in over 80% of the children, with subsequent decrease in their frequency of headaches using a dose of 1 mg/kg per day [58]. Owing to its side effects, especially its somnolence, this must be slowly titrated to this dose, typically over 8–12 weeks, increasing it by 0.25 mg/kg per day every 2 weeks or so.

Nortriptyline has sometimes been used to replace the amitriptyline due to the concern about its sedative side effect; however, it does raise the concern of increased arrhythmi,a and regular electrocardiograms may be required if nortriptyline is chosen.

Cyproheptadine, an antihistamine with antiserotonergic effects, has been used for the prevention of childhood headaches [59]. It may also have some calcium channel-blocking properties [60]. Historic studies have shown the effectiveness in small groups of children with a dosage range of 0.2–0.4 mg/kg per day. It tends to be well tolerated, with the most significant side effect being increased weight gain and sedation. Owing to the these adverse events, it tends to be limited to the younger children, with less usefulness in adolescents.

Beta blockers have been used for prevention of pediatric migraine [61, 62]. One of the original studies did demonstrate effectiveness, but follow-up studies have been more controversial. In the recent practice parameter, propranolol was noted to demonstrate a mixed responsiveness when used for pediatric migraine [29]. Furthermore, in children, the drop in blood pressure due to beta blockers, as well as exercise-induced asthma and potential depressive effects, limits its usefulness in this population.

Calcium channel blockers have been extensively studied in adults for headache prevention, but the data is lacking in the pediatric population except for flunarizine. Flunarizine is a calcium channel blocker available in Europe, but not in the USA. It has been demonstrated to be an effective migraine-preventive agent [63, 64]. In children in a double-blinded placebo-controlled crossover study, the baseline headache frequency was reduced in the flunarizine-treated group compared with placebo. The use of other calcium channel blockers may not be as effective and cannot be extrapolated. The one childhood study using nimodipine in a double-blinded placebo-controlled crossover study failed to demonstrate a significant difference between the placebo and active drug groups [65].

Prevention management of pediatric headaches may include some non-pharmaceutical treatments, including both riboflavin and coenzyme Q10 [66–69]. Their effectiveness and usefulness in children and adolescents has yet to be determined.

It is important in the use of preventative medications in this population to slowly titrate the dose to an effective level. Realistic expectations need to be addressed with the parent and patient, stating that it may take several weeks or months before an effective level and, therefore, an effective response is achieved. Sometimes, failure to respond to the preventative medication is due to inadequate management, either due to inadequate time of treatment or inadequate dosing. This can oftentimes be based on a patient's and parents' unrealistic expectations about the quickness with which they will respond to their treatment protocol. Educating the patient in the preventative therapy as in their acute therapy is essential to the patient's outcome.

Biobehavioral treatment

Biobehavioral therapy for pediatric headaches is felt to be essential to maintain a lifetime response to the treatment and management of headaches. Biobehavioral therapy can be divided into three components: treatment adherence, lifestyle management and psychological intervention, including biofeedback-assisted relaxation training.

Treatment adherence entails an understanding by the patient and parent about the importance of their treatment. Psychological or biobehavioral intervention may be useful in assisting with adherence by identifying obstacles to the medical plan and overcoming these barriers.

Biobehavioral therapy addresses adjustment of lifestyle habits. Many times, unhealthy lifestyle habits serve as a trigger for pediatric headaches: inadequate nutrition, skipping meals and altered sleep patterns. The importance of maintaining healthy lifestyle habits includes discussing the importance of adequate fluid hydration with limited use of caffeine, regular exercise, adequate nutrition with not skipping meals, and regular adequate sleep. Discussing with the parent and the patient that these are lifetime goals that will control the impact of migraine and minimize the use of medication may result in an overall long-term improvement in quality of life as well as potentially reverse any progressive nature of the disease.

Biofeedback-assisted relaxation therapy may be a useful addition. For children, single-session biofeedback-assisted relaxation therapy has been demonstrated to be learned quickly and effective in children as young as 9 years old [70–73].

8.3 Conclusions

The diagnostic criteria for pediatric migraine has improved, but continued improvements are necessary [11, 12]. Future work should focus on alternative case definitions based on behavior rather than symptoms. Exploring additional or alternative diagnostic features may be helpful. Presently, the ICHD-II criteria remain the best available reference gold standard [1].

Management options are improving for both children and adolescents with regard to the acute and preventive management of headache in general. The combined use of nonpharmacologic and pharmacologic modalities can prove to be quite efficacious in the complete relief of migraine in the pediatric population. A significant need remains for well-designed studies evaluating the efficacy and tolerability in the pediatric headache population.

References

1. Headache Classification Subcommittee of the International Headache Society (2004) The International Classification of Headache Disorders. *Cephalalgia: An International Journal of Headache*, **24**(Suppl. 1), 1–160.

2. Headache Classification Committee of the International Headache Society (1988) Classification and diagnostic criteria for headache disorders, cranial neuralgias and facial pain. *Cephalalgia: An International Journal of Headache*, **8**(Suppl 7), 1–96.

3. Gallai, V., Sarchielli, P., Carboni, F. *et al.* (1995) Applicability of the 1988 IHS criteria to headache patients under the age of 18 years attending 21 Italian headache clinics. *Headache*, **35**, 146–153.

4. Gladstein, J., Holden, E.W., Peralta, L. and Raven, M. (1993) Diagnoses and symptom patterns in children presenting to a pediatric headache clinic. *Headache*, **33**, 497–500.

5. Maytal, J., Young, M., Shechter, A. and Lipton, R.B. (1997) Pediatric migraine and the International Headache Society (IHS) criteria. *Neurology*, **48**, 602–607.

6. Mortimer, M.J., Kay, J. and Jaron, A. (1992) Epidemiology of headache and childhood migraine in an urban general practice using ad hoc, Vahlquist and IHS criteria. *Developmental Medicine and Child Neurology*, **34**, 1095–1101.

7. Seshia, S.S., Wolstin, J.R., Adams, C. *et al.* (1994) International Headache Society criteria and childhood headache. *Developmental Medicine and Child Neurology*, **36**, 419–428.

8. Wober-Bingol, C., Wober, C., Karwautz, A. *et al.* (1995) Diagnosis of headache in childhood and adolescence: a study in 437 patients. *Cephalalgia: An International Journal of Headache*, **15**(1), 13–21; discussion, 4.

9. Featherstone, H.J. (1985) Migraine and muscle contraction headaches: a continuum. *Headache*, **25**(4), 194–198.

10. Viswanathan, V., Bridges, S.J., Whitehouse, W. and Newton, R.W. (1998) Childhood headaches: discrete entities or continuum? *Developmental Medicine and Child Neurology*, **40**(8), 544–550.

11. Cady, R., Schreiber, C., Farmer, K. and Sheftell, F. (2002) Primary headaches: a convergence hypothesis. *Headache*, **42**, 204–216.

12. Lipton, R.B., Stewart, W.F., Cady, R. *et al.* (2000) Sumatriptan for the range of headaches in migraine sufferers: results of the Spectrum Study. *Headache*, **40**, 783–791.

13. Stewart, W.F., Shechter, A. and Lipton, R.B. (1994) Migraine heterogeneity. Disability, pain intensity, and attack frequency and duration. *Neurology*, **44**(6), (Suppl. 4), S24–S39.

14. Vahlquist, B. and Hackzell, G. (1949) Migraine of early onset. A study of thirty one cases in which the disease first appeared between one and four years of age. *Acta Paediatrica*, **38**, 622–636.

15. Bille, B. (1962) Migraine in school children. *Acta Paediatrica*, **51** (Suppl. 136), 16–151.

16. Friedman, A.P., Finley, K.H., Kunkle, E.C. *et al.* (1962) Classification of headache: Ad Hoc Committee on Classification of Headache. *The Journal of the American Medical Association*, **179**(9), 127–128.

17. Winner, P., Martinez, W., Mate, L. and Bello, L. (1995) Classification of pediatric migraine: proposed revisions to the IHS criteria. *Headache*, **35**, 407–410.

18. Winner, P., Wasiewski, W., Gladstein, J. and Linder, S. (1997) Multicenter prospective evaluation of proposed pediatric migraine revisions to the IHS criteria. *Headache*, **37**(9), 545–548.

19. Wobel-Bingol, C., Wober, C., Wagner-Ennsgraber, C. *et al.* (1996) IHS criteria and gender: a study on migraine and tension-type headache in children and adolescents. *Cephalalgia: An International Journal of Headache*, **16**, 107–112.

20. Metsahonkala, L. and Sillanpaa, M. (1994) Migraine in children – an evaluation of the IHS criteria. *Cephalalgia: An International Journal of Headache*, **14**(4), 285–290.

21. Lima, M.M., Padula, N.A., Santos, L.C. *et al.* (2005) Critical analysis of the international classification of headache disorders diagnostic criteria (ICHD I-1988) and (ICHD II-2004), for migraine in children and adolescents. *Cephalalgia: An International Journal of Headache*, **25**(11), 1042–1047.

22. Hershey, A.D., Winner, P., Kabbouche, M.A. *et al.* (2005) Use of the ICHD-II criteria in the diagnosis of pediatric migraine. *Headache*, **45**(10), 1288–1297.

23. Hershey, A.D., Powers, S.W., Vockell, A.L. *et al.* (2001) PedMIDAS: development of a questionnaire to assess disability of migraines in children. *Neurology*, **57**(11), 2034–2039.

24. Lewis, D.W., Rothner, A.D. and Linder, S.L. (2008) Evaluation of headache, in *Headaches in Children and Adolescents*, 2nd edn (eds P. Winner and A.D. Rothner), B.C. Decker, Inc., Hamilton, Ontario, pp. 19–35.

25. Lewis, D.W., Ashwal, S., Dahl, G. *et al.* (2002) Practice parameter: evaluation of children and adolescents with recurrent headaches: report of the Quality Standards Subcommittee of the American Academy of Neurology and the Practice Committee of the Child Neurology Society. *Neurology*, **59**(4), 490–498.

26. Varni, J.W., Seid, M. and Kurtin, P.S. (2001) PedsQL 4.0: reliability and validity of the Pediatric Quality of Life Inventory version 4.0 generic core scales in healthy and patient populations. *Medical Care*, **39**(8), 800–812.

27. Powers, S.W., Patton, S.R., Hommel, K.A. and Hershey, A.D. (2003) Quality of life in childhood migraines: clinical impact and comparison to other chronic illnesses. *Pediatrics*, **112**(1), (Pt 1), e1–e5.

28. Linder, S.L. (2005) Understanding the comprehensive pediatric headache examination. *Pediatric Annals*, **34**(6), 442–446.

29. Lewis, D., Ashwal, S., Hershey, A. *et al.* (2004) Practice Parameter: Pharmacological treatment of migraine headache in children and adolescents: Report of the American Academy of Neurology Quality Standards Subcommittee and the Practice Committee of the Child Neurology Society. *Neurology*, **63**(12), 2215–2224.

30. Hershey, A.D., Powers, S.W., Vockell, A.L. *et al.* (2004) Development of a patient-based grading scale for PedMIDAS. *Cephalalgia: An International Journal of Headache*, **24**(10), 844–849.

31. Hämäläinen, M.L., Hoppu, K., Valkeila, E. and Santavuori, P. (1997) Ibuprofen or acetaminophen for the acute treatment of migraine in children. *Neurology*, **48**, 103–107.

32. Lewis, D.W., Kellstein, D., Dahl, G. *et al.* (2002) Children's ibuprofen suspension for the acute treatment of pediatric migraine. *Headache*, **42**(8), 780–786.

33. Linder, S.L. (1995) Subcutaneous sumatriptan in the clinical setting: The first fifty consecutive patients with acute migraine in a pediatric neurology office practice. *Headache*, **35**, 291–292.

34. Winner, P., Prensky, A. and Linder, S. (1996) Efficacy and safety of oral sumatriptan in adolescent migraines. Presented at the American Association for the Study of Headache Chicago, IL.

35. Winner, P., Rothner, D., Saper, J. *et al.* (2000) A randomized, double-blind, placebo-controlled study of sumatriptan nasal spray in the treatment of acute migraine in adolescents. *Pediatrics*, **106**, 989–997.

36. Winner, P., Rothner, A.D., Wooen, J. *et al.* (2004) Randomized, double-blind, placebo-controlled study of sumatriptan nasal spray in adolescent migraineurs. *Neurology*, **62**, A182.

37. Winner, P., Lewis, D., Visser, W.H. *et al.* (2002) Rizatriptan 5 mg for the acute treatment of migraine in adolescents: a randomized, double-blind, placebo-controlled study. *Headache*, **42**(1), 49–55.

38. Linder, S.L. and Dowson, A.J. (2000) Zolmitriptan provides effective migraine relief in adolescents. *International Journal of Clinical Practice*, **54**(7), 466–469.

39. Lipton, R.B., Stewart, W.F., Stone, A.M. *et al.* (2000) Stratified care vs step care strategies for migraine: the Disability in Strategies of Care (DISC) Study: a randomized trial. *The Journal of the American Medical Association*, **284**(20), 2599–2605.

40. Smith, T.R., Sunshine, A., Stark, S.R. *et al.* (2005) Sumatriptan and naproxen sodium for the acute treatment of migraine. *Headache*, **45**(8), 983–991.

41. Linder, S.L. (1994) Treatment of childhood headache wtih dihydroergotamine mesylate. *Headache*, **34**, 578–580.

42. Jones, J., Sklar, D., Dougherty, J. and White, W. (1989) Randomized double-blind trial of intravenous prochlorperazine for the treatment of acute headache. *The Journal of the American Medical Association*, **261**, 1174–1176.

43. Peroutka, S.J. (1997) Dopamine and migraine. *Neurology*, **49**, 650–656.

44. Kabbouche, M.A., Vockell, A.L., LeCates, S.L. *et al.* (2001) Tolerability and effectiveness of prochlorperazine for intractable migraine in children. *Pediatrics*, **107**(4), E62.

45. Burstein, R. and Cutrer, F.M. (2000) The development of cutaneous allodynia during a migraine attack: clinical evidence for the sequential recruitment of spinal and supraspinal nociceptive neurons in migraine. *Brain: A Journal of Neurology*, **123**, 1703–1709.

46. Burstein, R., Collins, B. and Jakubowski, M. (2004) Defeating migraine pain with triptans: a race against the development of cutaneous allodynia. *Annals of Neurology*, **55**(1), 19–26.

47. Burstein, R. and Jakubowski, M. (2004) Analgesic triptan action in an animal model of intracranial pain: A race against the development of central sensitization. *Annals of Neurology*, **55**(1), 27–36.

48. Mathew, N.T., Saper, J.R., Silberstein, S.D. *et al.* (1995) Migraine prophylaxis with divalproex. *Archives of Neurology*, **52**, 281–286.

49. Silberstein, S.D. (1996) Divalproex sodium in headache: literature review and clinical guidelines. *Headache*, **36**(9), 547–555.

50. Caruso, J.M., Brown, W.D., Exil, G. and Gascon, G.G. (2000) The efficacy of divalproex sodium in the prophylactic treatment of children with migraine. *Headache*, **40**, 672–676.

51. Serdaroglu, G., Erhan, E., Tekgul, H. *et al.* (2002) Sodium valproate prophylaxis in childhood migraine. *Headache*, **42**(8), 819–822.

52. Hershey, A.D., Powers, S.W., Vockell, A.L. *et al.* (2002) Effectiveness of topiramate in the prevention of childhood headaches. *Headache*, **42**(8), 810–818.

53. Winner, P., Pearlman, E., Linder, S. *et al.* (2004) Topiramate for the prevention of migraines in children and adolescence: a randomized, double-blind, placebo-controlled trial. *Headache*, **44**, 481.

54. Couch, J.R., Ziegler, D.K. and Hassanein, R. (1976) Amitriptyline in the prophylaxis of migraine. Effectiveness and relationship of antimigraine and antidepressant effects. *Neurology*, **26**, 121–127.

55. Gomersall, J.D. and Stuart, A. (1973) Amitriptyline in migraine prophylaxis. *Journal of Neurology, Neurosurgery, and Psychiatry*, **36**, 684–690.

56. Couch, J.R. and Hassanein, R.S., (1979) Amitriptyline in migraine prophylaxis. *Archives of Neurology*, **36**, 695–699.

57. Levinstein, B. (1991) A comparative study of cyproheptadine, amitriptyline, and propranolol in the treatment of adolescent migraine. *Cephalalgia: An International Journal of Headache*, **11**, 122–123.

58. Hershey, A.D., Powers, S.W., Bentti, A.L. and Degrauw, T.J. (2000) Effectiveness of amitriptyline in the prophylactic management of childhood headaches. *Headache*, **40**(7), 539–549.

59. Bille, B., Ludvigsson, J. and Sanner, G. (1977) Prophylaxis of migraine in children. *Headache*, **17**, 61–63.

60. Peroutka, S.J. and Allen, G.S. (1984) The calcium antagonist properties of cyproheptadine: implications for antimigraine action. *Neurology*, **34**(3), 304–309.

61. Ludvigsson, J. (1974) Propranolol used in prophylaxis of migraine in children. *Acta Neurologica Scandinavica*, **50**, 109–115.

62. Ziegler, D.K. and Hurwitz, A. (1993) Propranolol and amitriptyline in prophylaxis of migraine. *Archives of Neurology*, **50**, 825–830.

63. Sorge, F., De Simone, R., Marano, E. *et al.* (1988) Flunarizine in prophylaxis of childhood migraine. A double-blind, placebo-controlled, crossover study. *Cephalalgia: An International Journal of Headache*, **8**(1), 1–6.

64. Guidetti, V., Moscato, D., Ottaviano, S. *et al.* (1987) Flunarizine and migraine in childhood. An evaluation of endocrine function. *Cephalalgia: An International Journal of Headache*, **7**(4), 263–266.

65. Battistella, P.A., Ruffilli, R., Moro, R. *et al.* (1990) A placebo-controlled crossover trial of nimodipine in pediatric migraine. *Headache*, **30**(5), 264–268.

66. Schoenen, J., Jacquy, J. and Lenaerts, M. (1998) Effectiveness of high-dose riboflavin in migraine prophylaxis: a randomized controlled trial. *Neurology*, **50**, 466–470.

67. Boehnke, C., Reuter, U., Flach, U. *et al.* (2004) High-dose riboflavin treatment is efficacious in migraine prophylaxis: an open study in a tertiary care centre. *European Journal of Neurology*, **11**(7), 475–477.

68. Rozen, T.D., Oshinsky, M.L., Gebeline, C.A. *et al.* (2002) Open label trial of coenzyme Q10 as a migraine preventive. *Cephalalgia: An International Journal of Headache*, **22**(2), 137–141.

69. Sandor, P.S., Di Clemente, L., Coppola, G. *et al.* (2005) Efficacy of coenzyme Q10 in migraine prophylaxis: a randomized controlled trial. *Neurology*, **64**(4), 713–715.

70. Daly, E., Donn, P., Galliher, M. and Zimmerman, J. (1983) Biofeedback applications to migraine and tension headaches: A double-blinded outcome study. *Biofeedback and Self-Regulation*, **8**(1), 135–152.

71. Werder, D. and Sargent, J. (1984) A study of childhood headache using biofeedback as a treatment alternative. *Headache*, **24**, 122–126.

72. Powers, S.W. and Spirito, A. (1998) *Biofeedback*, John Wiley & Sons, Inc., New York.

73. Powers, S.W. and Hershey, A.D. (2002) Biofeedback for childhood migraine, in *Current Management in Child Neurology*, 2nd edn (ed. B.L. Maria), B.C. Decker, Inc., Hamilton, Ontario, pp. 83–85.

9
Childhood periodic syndromes

Marielle A. Kabbouche

Migraine is a well-defined disease with symptoms carried from childhood into adult life [1, 2]. Migraine often presents as a paroxysmal syndrome with periodic attacks and associated symptoms, these attacks occurring at variable frequency and duration.

Multiple other periodic syndromes have been frequently described in children, with some of them sharing close symptomatology with migraine, especially a future occurrence of migraine in these children, which favored the term of 'migraine equivalents' for these clinical syndromes. These periodic syndromes are most probably precursors for migraine, and their diagnosis may be a flag for the development of migraine later in life.

In this chapter we will be reviewing these periodic syndromes: their clinical picture, how to diagnose them, necessary testing, differential diagnosis to contemplate, their future outcome and available therapies.

Periodic syndromes of childhood and migraine equivalents in childhood include [3]:

1. benign paroxysmal vertigo (BPV);

2. abdominal migraine (AM);

3. cyclical vomiting syndrome (CVS);

4. alternating hemiplegia of childhood (AHC);

Pediatric Headaches in Clinical Practice   Andrew D. Hershey, Paul Winner, Marielle A. Kabbouche and Scott W. Powers
© 2009 John Wiley & Sons, Ltd.

5. benign paroxysmal torticolis (BPT);

6. others – motion/car sickness; sleep disturbances – night terrors, sleep walking, sleep talking, recurrent unexplained fever.

The three syndromes that are recognized by International Classification of Headache Disorders II (ICHD-II) as precursors of migraine headache are BPV, AM and CVS [4].

9.1 BPV: Benign paroxysmal vertigo

BPV is primarily a disorder of infants and preschool children, but it still can occur in older children with variation of age between 3 months and 8 years [5–7].

Clinical features

BPV is described as recurrent attacks of sudden vertigo that is maximal at onset; ataxia may be present but rare. The vertigo is so severe that standing may be impossible. The child looks frightened and wants to be held by his care giver. A transient decrease in vestibular function may be noticed, but *consciousness is maintained* throughout the event. Headache is not usually part of the clinical picture. The attacks may last a few minutes and in extreme cases hours to 2 days. Their frequency varies from a few episodes a week to once a year and may ease in a few months to a few years before they disappear spontaneously. Children should have a normal vestibular function between attacks with no residual symptoms.

The main symptoms of BPV are:

– pallor;

– nystagmus;

– fear;

– rarely other symptoms, such as sweating and vomiting;

– consciousness is *always* preserved.

The ICHD-II defines BPV as shown in Table 9.1.

Table 9.1   ICHD-II definition of BPV (ICHD-II criteria reproduced with permission from Blackwell Publishing)

A	At least five attacks fulfilling criterion (B–D).
B	Multiple episodes of severe vertigo occurring without warning and resolving spontaneously after minutes or hours.
C	Normal neurological examination and audiometric/vestibular functions between attacks.
D	Normal electroencephalogram.

Differential diagnosis

The diagnosis of the syndrome is mostly a clinical diagnosis through a *detailed history* on the onset of the attacks, duration, frequency, associated symptoms, family history (40% of the children will have a positive family history of migraine) and a *detailed physical examination* (general and neurological).

Testing is only useful to exclude other diagnoses, such as:

1. posterior fossa tumors;

2. seizure/epilepsy;

3. vestibular problems.

It is recommended to undertake the following tests at the initial visit:

- brain imaging, preferably by magnetic resonance imaging (MRI), to have a clear view of the posterior fossa;

- an electroencephalogram (EEG), to evaluate the possibility of seizures that can have a similar clinical picture;

- audiometric and vestibular function, the latter to be done between attacks.

Outcome

Nineteen patients were followed long term by Lindskog *et al.* [8] after they were diagnosed. The age of onset of BPV was 5 months to 8 years. The resolution of the symptoms occurred 3 months to 8 years post-evaluation. Follow-ups made

13–20 years later revealed that 21% developed typical migraine headache and all were BPV free.

Treatment

Parents should first be educated about the benign form and the outcome of the symptoms, since the clinical picture may be stressful to them. They should understand that the testing is not done due to the complexity of BPV, but rather to eliminate other rare diseases.

Medical treatment is often unnecessary if the episodes are brief and not frequent. Education about healthy habits should be emphasized, including regular diet, sleep and hydration.

If the episodes become more frequent or are lasting longer, then preventive medications can be introduced and at this age cyproheptadine may be one of the first choices. Preventive medications are to be titrated gradually over a few weeks and may not be effective until the full dose is reached. Acute therapy may not be beneficial if the spell is lasting a few minutes, but if lasting 15 min or longer then a nonsteroidal analgesic may be introduced at onset of the attack, such as ibuprofen at 10 mg/kg with hydrating fluids.

9.2 AM: Abdominal migraine

Chronic recurrent abdominal pain is frequent in childhood [9–11]. This entity is classified by the American Academy of Pediatrics and the North American Society of Pediatric Gastroenterology, Hepatology and Nutrition as follows:

– chronic abdominal pain;

– functional abdominal pain;

– functional dyspepsia;

– irritable bowel syndrome;

– abdominal migraine;

– functional abdominal pain syndrome.

AM was added to the classification due to the strong association of headache in the symptomatology. Ramchandani *et al.* [9] describe in their review that, by the age of 6 years, 55.4% of children with recurrent abdominal pain will have complained of headache.

Clinical features

AM is a syndrome characterized by episodes of recurrent moderate to severe abdominal pain that often is associated with nausea and sometimes with vomiting. The pain is so strong that it interferes with normal daily activities. The episodes are separated by periods of good health and wellness.

The syndrome often occurs between the ages of 5 and 9 years; but extremes can be seen, with children affected very early in life and in adulthood. Most children affected have a strong family history of migraine with or without aura and eventually they will develop migraine headache.

The main symptoms of AM are:

- recurrent moderate to severe abdominal pain;

- nausea- anorexia;

- sometimes vomiting;

- the pain interferes with regular daily activities;

- pallor.

There is no diagnostic test to confirm AM; the diagnosis relies on a detailed history of the episodes, family history, and detailed physical and neurological examinations. AM is a diagnosis of exclusion, and other diagnoses should be considered and eliminated first.

The ICHD-II defines AM as an idiopathic recurrent disorder seen mainly in children and characterized by episodic midline abdominal pain manifesting in attacks lasting 1–72 h with normality between episodes. The pain is of moderate to severe intensity and associated with vasomotor symptoms, nausea and vomiting.

Diagnostic criteria

The AM diagnostic criteria are given in Table 9.2.

Differential diagnosis

Diagnoses to be considered prior to considering the diagnosis of AM are given in Table 9.3.

The recommendations are to have a full evaluation to rule out all the possibilities in Table 9.3, including a referral to specialty clinics, as well as brain imaging (preferably an MRI scan) and an EEG in case of alteration of consciousness.

Table 9.2 AM diagnostic criteria

A. At least five attacks fulfilling criteria B–D.
B. Attacks of abdominal pain lasting 1–72 h (untreated or unsuccessfully treated).
C. Abdominal pain has all of the following characteristics:
   1. midline location, periumbilical or poorly localized;
   2. dull or 'just sore' quality;
   3. moderate or severe intensity.
D. During abdominal pain at least two of the following:
   1. anorexia;
   2. nausea;
   3. vomiting;
   4. pallor.
E. Not attributed to another disorder.

Note
1.   In particular, history and physical examination do not show signs of gastrointestinal or renal disease or such disease has been ruled out by appropriate investigations.

Comments
Pain is severe enough to interfere with normal daily activities. Children may find it difficult to distinguish anorexia from nausea. The pallor is often accompanied by dark shadows under the eyes. In a few patients flushing is the predominant vasomotor phenomenon. Most children with abdominal migraine will develop migraine headache later in life.

Table 9.3 Diagnoses to be considered prior to considering diagnosis of AM

Gastrointestinal problems, including:
1. peptic ulcer disease;
2. cholecystitis;
3. gastroesophageal reflux;
4. gastrointestinal obstruction especially duodenal due to the location of the pain;
5. Crohn's disease;
6. irritable bowel syndrome;
7. other.

Urogenital disorders

Central nervous system involvement
1. Posterior fossa tumor if nausea and vomiting are predominant.
2. Seizures and epilepsy if the abdominal pain is associated with an alteration of consciousness.

Outcome

Prognosis of childhood AM was studied by Dignan *et al.* [12]. Fifty-four children with the diagnosis of AM were followed at 7–10 years after their first evaluation:

- 61% had a resolution of the AM;

- 72% of the previously diagnosed AM are currently (52%) or previously (18%) suffering from migraine headache compared with only 20% of the controlled group.

These results not only show the outcome of AM, but also support the concept of AM being a precursor of migraine with or without aura.

Treatment

Migraine therapy is effective in treating most AM [13]. As for other forms of migraine, acute and preventive medications are used depending on the clinical picture.

For infrequent attacks, acute medications such as nonsteroidal anti-inflammatory drugs, antinausea medications and triptan are effective when used at onset of symptoms. The choice of medicine depends on the age of the patient, as well as on other associated comorbidities.

For frequent episodes, a preventive therapy should be added. The use of preventive medicine also depends on the age of the patient and associated comorbidities. Any preventive medication used for migraine prophylaxis can be explored and given the time to be tapered to an appropriate dose for best efficacy.

Healthy habits are to be emphasized, including regular meals, hydration, good sleep and exercise.

9.3 CVS: Cyclical vomiting syndrome

Clinical features

The original description in 1882 of cyclic vomiting is very useful today: 'fits of vomiting with disease-free intervals' [14].

CVS is clinically defined as violent intractable frequent episodes of vomiting lasting hours to days. It is a complex syndrome that occurs mostly in infants and children and is less common in adults. The episodes of vomiting are often accompanied by dehydration. Between the attacks children regain their normal health and function. Headache is not usually part of the symptoms. Most of the attacks are precipitated by infection, menstruation, physical or mental stress. They can be predicted, occurring regularly at intervals of a few months. The dehydration may be so severe that intravenous (IV) hydration and correction of the electrolytes imbalance is needed in an inpatient setting. Cases of central nervous system venous thrombosis can be seen in these cases of severe hydration, especially in younger children.

Cyclic vomiting is thought to be the result of abnormal activity in the area postrema.

The diagnosis of CVS is a diagnosis of exclusion, and other pathologies should be entertained prior to making the final decision.

The ICHD-II defines CVS as shown in Table 9.4.

Table 9.4 ICHD-II definition of CVS (ICHD-II criteria reproduced with permission from Blackwell Publishing)

Description
Recurrent episodic attacks, usually stereotypical in the individual patient, of vomiting and intense nausea. Attacks are associated with pallor and lethargy. There is complete resolution of symptoms between attacks.

Diagnostic criteria
A.   At least five attacks fulfilling criteria band C.
B.   Episodic attacks, stereotypical in the individual patient, of intense nausea and vomiting lasting from 1 h to 5 days.
C.   Vomiting during attacks occurs at least four times per hour for at least 1 h.
D.   Symptom free between attacks
E.   Not attributed to another disorder.[1]

Note
1.   In particular, history and physical examination do not show signs of gastrointestinal disease.

Comment
Cyclical vomiting is a self-limiting episodic condition of childhood, with periods of complete normality between episodes. This disorder was not included as a childhood periodic syndrome in the first edition of *The International Classification of Headache Disorders*. The clinical features of this syndrome resemble those found in association with migraine headaches, and multiple threads of research over recent years have suggested that cyclical vomiting is a condition related to migraine.

Differential diagnosis

As mentioned in the definition, cyclic vomiting is a diagnosis of exclusion. Other pathologies need to be contemplated prior to the final decision. The differential diagnoses include, but are not limited to:

1. gastrointestinal disorders – gastroesophageal reflux, bowel obstruction;

2. central nervous system neoplasm;

3. metabolic disorders.

The initial evaluation should include a work-up by a pediatric gastroenterology service, an MRI scan of the brain, a full evaluation including a complete blood count with differential, fasting glucose, renal/electrolytes/ liver profile, and a baseline metabolic profile (plasma aminoacids, urine organic acids, ammonia level, plasma pyruvate and lactate).

Outcome

Fitzpatrick *et al.* [15] published data on a 10-year follow-up study for CVS: 50 children were diagnosed with CVS, 41 participated in the follow-up data.
Age varied as follows:

age of onset of CVS, 5.8 ± 3.3 years;

age of diagnosis, 8.2 ± 3.5 years;

age at follow up, 12.8 ± 4.8 years.

The follow-up data revealed that 61% of the patients had a resolution of cyclic vomiting, with 39% occurring early; 42% had headaches and migraine at follow up; 37% had chronic abdominal pain.

It is clear from these results that even if the attacks of cyclic vomiting subside, children are still left with other symptoms that still need close attention.

Treatment

David R. Fleisher, MD, describes the attack as a stepwise clinical picture [16]. The phases of the attack are then divided and treated gradually, depending on the symptomatology of the specific phase.

Phase 1: the nausea-free interval between episodes. Patients are symptom free, healthy. If their attacks are frequent usually and disabling, then migraine prophylaxis should be started to decrease the severity and the frequency of the attacks. The preventive therapy should consider the age of the patient, associated comorbidities and toxicities. In addition, it is helpful during this calm phase to identify and ameliorate conditions that may predispose to or trigger episodes, such as chronic sinusitis/infections, clinically significant anxiety, premenstrual symptoms, motion sickness or metabolic stress (e.g. prolonged caloric deprivation in patients who may have a defect in fatty acid oxidation). Education of the patient and family is always a key for success in treating headache, migraine and their variants. The family and patient should be educated about healthy habits, and this phase is the best time to do it.

Phase 2: the prodrome. This is the interval that starts when the patient begins to feel symptoms signaling the approach of an episode, but is still able to retain oral medications. It ends with the onset of vomiting. The prodrome might last days, minutes, or may not occur at all in patients who wake from sleep already vomiting. Nausea may be the prominent symptom and should be treated with antinausea medicine and oral hydration. Anxiety may be at its peak, since the patient is already aware that the worst is yet to come. Lorazepam has been successfully used to help control the anxiety, some of the nausea and induces sleep. For *nausea*, try ondansetron (*Zofran*) liquid, tablets or oral disintegrating tablets at 0.3–0.4 mg/kg per dose. (This is twice the dose recommended for chemotherapy patients.) *Anxiety* potentiates nausea. Lorazepam (*Ativan*) is anxiolytic, antiemetic and promotes sleep. It works well together with ondansetron. Lorazepam tablets are almost tasteless and dissolve in the mouth without the patient having to drink. For associated *AM*, try *ibuprofen* p.o. 10 mg/kg. Triptans can be effective and can be initiated at the start of this phase, including the tablets, nasal sprays and injectables.

Phase 3: the attack itself. This is characterized by intractable nausea and vomiting. Patients who writhe and moan between bouts of vomiting have intense abdominal ache and/or severe retrosternal pain.

The possible acute complications of untreated episodes include hypovolemic shock, electrolyte depletion, tetany, hematemesis and secretion of inappropriate antidiuretic hormone (SIADH). The nausea of CVS episodes is agonizing. Therefore, treatment of CVS episodes must be prompt. If treatment is delayed, the patient's extreme distress predisposes them to fear the next episode, and, since anticipatory anxiety can cause nausea, their fear may cause more frequent attacks. Most of these episodes will need admission to an emergency room or hospital bed for aggressive hydration.

To treat phase 3, cannulate a vein, draw whatever diagnostic blood samples are necessary, consider the need for a normal saline bolus and start maintenance IV fluids. If the possibility of an underlying metabolic defect, such as medium-chain acyl-CoA dehydrogenase, has not been ruled out, then the IV fluid should contain *10% glucose* during the first 24 h; the response or lack of response to IV glucose has diagnostic and therapeutic implications. Otherwise, *5% dextrose in 0.5 N saline with KCl and an H-2 blocker* can be used for IV fluid maintenance.

As soon as IV access is established, attempt to *terminate* the episode by giving *lorazepam* by slow IV push (0.05–0.1 mg/kg, maximum 3 mg per dose) and ondansetron (*Zofran*) at 0.3–0.4 mg/kg per dose by IV piggyback over 15 min. The patient will respond in one of three ways: (1) the nausea clears and does not return; (2) the nausea clears, but returns within minutes or hours; or (3) the nausea does not clear.

In the first case, cap or remove the IV, give 4–8 mg p.o. of ondansetron and send the patient home. In the second and third cases, termination has failed and there is no way to give relief other than to *sedate* the patient. The brain, not the gastrointestinal tract, is the origin of cyclic vomiting and sleep stops such vomiting. It also makes patients unaware of their nausea, giving them an escape from what would otherwise be relentless misery. Preferred sedative drugs are nonaddictive and nonemetogenic: *chlorpromazine* (0.5–1 mg/kg per dose) with diphenhydramine (0.5–1 mg/kg per dose) in 50 ml of normal saline and infuse over 15 min. This combination of sedatives should be repeated as needed for wakefulness with nausea, as often as 3–4 h for as long as the episode lasts. DO NOT USE CHLORPROMAZINE UNTIL HYPOVOLEMIA HAS BEEN CORRECTED to avoid hypotension.

Hematemesis is common. It is often due to 'prolapse gastropathy', in which there is bleeding of the mucosa of the proximal stomach as intense retching forces the cardia up into the lower esophagus where it is squeezed and bruised. Although hematemesis of this type seldom causes serious blood loss, it does not preclude bleeding from the esophageal mucosa or from Mallory–Weiss tears.

Monitor the pH of vomitus. If it remains below 4.5, increase the IV dose of H-2 blocker.

Intense nausea may be accompanied by SIADH. Monitor urine specific gravity; if it remains high in the presence of adequate hydration, then check for low serum osmolality and hyponatremia and restrict water input until laboratory values return to normal.

Many patients experience intense thirst, which compels them to drink even though they know it will come back up almost immediately. If compulsive drinking is followed by self-induced vomiting during episodes, do not mistake this behavior for bulimia! Drinking dilutes acid and bile, thereby making the vomitus less of a contact irritant to the esophagus and mouth. Emesis can be induced more easily from a full stomach than an empty one. The transient lessening of nausea that follows self-induced vomiting makes this comfort-seeking behavior worth the trouble for some patients. Keeping the patient n.p.o. is almost impossible. Sedation eliminates the drink-and-vomit behavior.

Phase 4: the recovery phase. This begins when vomiting is over and the nausea begins to subside. It ends when the patient's appetite, tolerance for food and vigor become normal. Recovery tends to be prolonged when inadequate management of the episode permitted severe fluid and electrolyte deficits and marked weight loss [17, 18].

9.4 AHC: Alternating hemiplegia of childhood

Clinical features

AHC is characterized by episodes of hemiparesis, monoparesis or quadrepar-esis [19]. These episodes can be associated with involuntary movements (dystonia, choreoathetosis, etc.). The onset of the episodes is at a very young age and over time may demonstrate a gradual occurrence of developmental delay.

ACH is considered a chronic progressive disorder with high prevalence of neurological deficit.

It is distinguished from familial hemiplegic migraine by its infantile onset and by its characteristic associated symptoms [20]. The disease usually occurs before 18 months of age (mean age of 8 months) and is associated with headache, alternating hemiplegia, altered consciousness, movement disorders such as choreoathetosis and dystonia, ocular palsies and nystagmus, autonomic dys-function and progressive mental retardation. The duration of the attack varies between minutes and days, and the intensity waxes and wanes during each episode. During a prolonged episode the hemiplegia may shift from one side to another; both sides may be affected. The specific picture is that the hemiplegia disappears during sleep.

The ICHD-II diagnostic criteria of AHC are shown in Table 9.5.

Table 9.5   ICHD-II diagnostic criteria of AHC (ICHD-II criteria reproduced with permission from Blackwell Publishing)

A.   Recurrent attacks of hemiplegia alternating between the two sides of the body.
B.   Onset before the age of 18 months.
C.   At least one other paroxysmal phenomenon is associated with the bouts of hemiplegia or occurs independently, such as: tonic spells, dystonic posturing, choreoathetoid movements, nystagmus or other ocular motor abnormalities, autonomic disturbances.
D.   Evidence of mental and/or neurological deficit(s).
E.   Not attributed to another disorder.

Differential diagnosis

- Hemiplegic migraine;

- Moyamoya disease;

- Alper disease;

- mitochondrial disease.

Any infant with a clinical picture of alternating hemiplegia before deciding on the final diagnosis of AHC should go through a full work-up, including imaging of the brain with an MRI scan/magnetic resonance angiography to evaluate any vascular/structural abnormality in the brain, thrombotic evaluation, an EEG to evaluate for seizures and a full mitochondrial evaluation.

Outcome

This migraine variant is a sporadic progressive neurological disorder It is thought to be a mitochondrial disorder, some families show mutations in a sodium potassium adenosine triphosphahtase (ATPase).

Stepwise neurological impairment occurs due to lack of complete recovery from individual attacks.

Treatment

Most migraine preventive therapies has not been very successful. Except for flunarizine. Flunarizine is a calcium channel blocker that can decrease the frequency and severity of the attacks.

9.5 BPT: Benign paroxysmal torticolis

Clinical features

BPT may be a variant of basilar migraine or be closely related to BPV. Onset is always in the first year of age. It is characterized by a head tilt (not always to the same side for each attack), vomiting and ataxia lasting hours to days. Some children may only have the torticolis; others will have the full-blown syndrome. The attacks last between 1 and 3 days and always resolves spontaneously. The episodes can occur multiple times a year. Often, a family history of migraine is present. It can gradually evolve into a typical migraine headache with or without aura later. No specific evaluation is necessary; the diagnosis is a clinical diagnosis. The history and full detailed general and neurological examination arc cnough to get to the final diagnosis.

A differential diagnosis should still be entertained due to the usual very young age of the presenting patient.

The differential diagnoses include posterior fossa abnormalities, cervical spine abnormalities and seizures.

An MRI of the brain as well as the cervical spine are recommended to evaluate any possible structural abnormality; an EEG should be taken to rule out any seizure.

The ICHD-II defines BPT as shown in Table 9.6.

Outcome

With time, the attacks may evolve into a classical migraine headache with or without aura, or into episodes characteristic of BPV. They may also cease without any further symptomatology.

Table 9.6 ICHD-II (A1.3.5) definition of BPT (ICHD-II criteria reproduced with permission from Blackwell Publishing)

A. Episodic attacks, in a young child, with all of the following characteristics and fulfilling criterion B:
   tilt of the head to one side (not always the same side), with or without slight rotation, lasting minutes to days, remitting spontaneously and tending to recur monthly.

B. During attacks, symptoms and/or signs of one or more of the following:
   pallor;
   irritability;
   malaise;
   vomiting;
   ataxia.

C. Normal neurological examination between attacks.

D. Not attributed to another disorder.

Treatment

The acute attacks usually do not affect the child. Migraine medications may be necessary if the episodes are prolonged or frequent.

References

1. Bille, B. (1991) Migraine in childhood and its prognosis. *Cephalalgia: An International Journal of Headache*, **1**, 71–75.

2. Bille, B. (1997) A 40-year follow-up of school children with migraine. *Cephalalgia: An International Journal of Headache*, **17**, 488–491.

3. Al-Twaijri, W.A. and Shevell, M.I. (2002) Pediatric migraine equivalents: occurrence and clinical features in practice. *Pediatric Neurology*, **26**, 365–368.

4. Headache Classification Subcommittee of the International Headache Society (2004) The International Classification of Headache Disorders: 2nd edition. *Cephalalgia*, **24** (Suppl 1), 1–160.

5. Fenichel, G.M. (1967) Migraine as a cause of benign paroxysmal vertigo of childhood. *The Journal of Pediatrics*, **71**, 114–115.

6. Dunn, D.W. and Snyder, C.H. (1976) Benign paroxysmal vertigo of childhood. *American Journal of Diseases of Children*, **130**, 1099–1100.

7. Drigo, P., Carli, G. and Laverda, A.M. (2001) Benign paroxysmal vertigo of childhood. *Brain & Development*, **23**, 38–41.

8. Lindskog, U., Odkvist, L., Noaksson, L. and Wallquist, J. (1999) Benign paroxysmal vertigo in childhood: a long-term follow-up. *Headache*, **39**(1), 33–37.

9. Ramchandani, P.G., Hotopf, M., Sandhu, B. *et al.* (2005) The epidemiology of recurrent abdominal pain from 2 to 6 years of age: results of a large, population-based study. *Pediatrics*, **116**(1), 46–50.

10. Farquar, H.A. (1956) Abdominal migraine in children. *BMJ (Clinical Research)*, **i**, 1082–1085.

11. Abu-Arafeh, I. and Russel, G. (1995) Prevalence and clinical features of abdominal migraine compared with those of migraine headache. *Archives of Disease in Childhood*, **72**, 413–417.

12. Dignan, F., Abu-Arafeh, I. and Russell, G. (2001) The prognosis of childhood abdominal migraine. *Archives of Disease in Childhood*, **84**, 415–418.

13. Russell, G., Abu-Arafeh, I. and Symon, D.N., (2002) Abdominal migraine: evidence for existence and treatment options. *Paediatric Drugs*, **4**, 1–8.

14. Li, B.U. (2001) Cyclic vomiting syndrome: age-old syndrome and new insights. *Seminars in Pediatric Neurology*, **8**, 13–21.

15. Fitzpatrick, E., Bourke, B., Drumm, B. and Rowland, M. (2008) The incidence of cyclic vomiting syndrome in children: population-based study. *American Journal of Gastroenterology*, **103** (4), 991–995.

16. Fleisher, D.R. (1999) Cyclic vomiting syndrome and migraine. *The Journal of Pediatrics*, **134**, 533–535.

17. Rashed, H., Abell, T.L., Familoni, B.O. *et al.* (1999) Autonomic function in cyclic vomiting syndrome and classic migraine. *Digestive Diseases and Sciences*, **44**(8) (8 Suppl 1), 74S–78S.

18. Welch, K.M. (1999) Scientific basis of migraine: speculation on the relationship to cyclic vomiting. *Digestive Diseases and Sciences*, **44**(8) (Suppl 1), 26–30.

19. Haan, J., Terwindt, G.M. and Ferrari, M.D. (1997) Genetics of migraine. *Neurologic Clinics*, **15**, 43–60.

20. Thomsen, L.L., Ostergaard, E., Olesen, J. and Russell, M.B. (2003) Evidence for a separate type of migraine with aura: sporadic hemiplegic migraine. *Neurology*, **60**, 595–601.

10

Tension-type headache: diagnosis and treatment

Andrew D. Hershey

In pediatric tertiary headache practices, migraine is the most common primary headache disorder managed, while the other primary headache disorders are much less frequently referred for headache specialty care. For tension-type headaches (TTHs) this may be due to the less severe nature of the headache pain and the lower disability. In the general population, however, TTH may be as frequent as, if not more frequent than, migraine. As a mild to moderate headache, it can often be managed without medical intervention and, therefore, may be easier to ignore. Conversely, the associated symptoms of migraine, especially vomiting, and the higher disability of migraine with subsequent restriction of school, family and social activities often raise concerns in the family and are brought to medical attention. TTHs, on the other hand, lack significant associated symptoms, are less severe and have less of an impact on disability, thus decreasing the likelihood of the child telling the parent and the parent seeking medical assistance.

10.1 Diagnosis of tension-type headaches (TTHs)

TTHs are generally thought of as mild recurrent headaches. Other names for this type of headache have included muscle contraction headache, idiopathic headache and tension headache. They can be infrequent (less than one a month), frequent (more than once a month, but not more than half the

Pediatric Headaches in Clinical Practice   Andrew D. Hershey, Paul Winner, Marielle A. Kabbouche and Scott W. Powers
© 2009 John Wiley & Sons, Ltd.

month) and chronic (more than half the month). The headache severity is usually described as mild to moderate with the location being diffuse or in a band-like pattern and having a pressing pain quality. As a primary headache disorder, no secondary etiologies should be identified and the patient should have a normal neurological examination and comprehensive headache examination. As a primary headache, the most difficult component of making the diagnosis of TTH is separating it from migraine. This is largely due to the overlapping diagnostic characteristics, especially in severity (TTH as mild to moderate; migraine as moderate to severe) and associated symptoms (the allowance of nausea, photophobia or phonophobia in TTH, but not vomiting).

The International Classification of Headache Disorders, 2nd Edition (ICHD-II) [1] identifies four subtypes of TTH: 2.1 Infrequent episodic tension-type headache, 2.2 Frequent episodic tension-type headache, 2.3 Chronic tension-type headache and 2.4 Probable tension-type headache. These are further subclassified according to the presence or absence of pericranial tenderness.

As in diagnosing any of the primary headache disorders in children (Chapters 2 and 3), establishing a diagnosis of TTH in children is often difficult due to a lack of recognition of the headache characteristics, either due to a misunderstanding of the questions asked by the interviewer or separating the features from migraine. This may be heightened in TTH due to the lack of disease impact and disability, such that the patient and parent may not attend to these features as readily as they do for migraine.

Frequently, the patient and parent may be vague in their descriptions, making the headache seem more TTH like, when in fact it may be migraine. Using standardized criteria such as the ICHD-II criteria is useful in the diagnosis of pediatric headaches and can serve to guide the interview process. Children's headache diagnosis is further complicated by being shorter in duration with spontaneous resolution or response to rest, sleep or behavioral therapies. Owing to these issues, it may be necessary to observe the child over time and utilize diaries to identify the diagnostic characteristics.

The typical features that separate TTH (Table 10.1) from migraine are a lack of throbbing or pulsatile quality of the pain, a diffuse location, a mild severity and lack of significant associated symptoms. Some researchers have argued that TTH and migraine are in a continuum [2], while others have argued that these are separate diseases with a broad spectrum of headaches represented by migraine [3]. Until biomarkers are available, this debate and the diagnosis of these two primary disorders will continue to have an overlapping difficulty.

Table 10.1 ICHD-II criteria. (Reproduced with permission from Blackwell Publishing)

Clinical Features
Infrequent TTH
A. At least 10 episodes occurring on <1 day per month on average (<12 days per year) and fulfilling criteria B–D
B. Headache lasting from 30 min to 7 days
C. Headache has at least two of the following characteristics:
    1. bilateral location
    2. pressing/tightening (nonpulsating) quality
    3. mild or moderate intensity
    4. not aggravated by routine physical activity such as walking or climbing stairs
D. Both of the following:
    1. no nausea or vomiting (anorexia may occur)
    2. no more than one of photophobia or phonophobia
E. Not attributed to another disorder

Frequent episodic TTH
A. At least 10 episodes occurring on ≥1 day but <15 days per month for at least 3 months (≥12 and <180 days per year) and fulfilling criteria B–D
B. Headache lasting from 30 min to 7 days
C. Headache has at least two of the following characteristics:
    1. bilateral location
    2. pressing/tightening (nonpulsating) quality
    3. mild or moderate intensity
    4. not aggravated by routine physical activity such as walking or climbing stairs
D. Both of the following:
    1. no nausea or vomiting (anorexia may occur)
    2. no more than one of photophobia or phonophobia
E. Not attributed to another disorder

Chronic TTH
Diagnostic criteria
A. Headache occurring on ≥15 days per month on average for >3 months (≥180 days per year) and fulfilling criteria B–D
B. Headache lasts hours or may be continuous
C. Headache has at least two of the following characteristics:
    1. bilateral location
    2. pressing/tightening (no-pulsating) quality
    3. mild or moderate intensity
    4. not aggravated by routine physical activity such as walking or climbing stairs
D. Both of the following:
    1. no more than one of photophobia, phonophobia or mild nausea
    2. neither moderate or severe nausea nor vomiting
E. Not attributed to another disorder

10.2 Epidemiology

In adults, TTHs are thought to be the most common type of primary headache disorder, with a lifetime prevalence ranging from 30 to 78%. Yet, TTHs remain the least well studied of the primary headache disorders. This is likely due to their low severity and lack of impact on a patient's quality of life and disability.

In children, all headache disorders have been less well studied, and this is especially true for TTH (reviewed by Anttila [4]). Epidemiology studies of TTH in children have been variable and have ranged from 0.9% [5] to 73% [6], with the most frequent range reported as 10–25% [4]. Using ICHD-I criteria, TTHs are reported in 9.8% of 7–16-year-olds in Sweden [7] and 12% of 12-year-olds in Finland [8]. In the study from Sweden, the prevalence of TTH increased with age; and if the requirements for recurrent headaches and duration were excluded, the prevalence reached 23%. In the study from Finland, many of the children diagnosed with TTH had migrainous features. Muscle tenderness was not a characteristic of TTH in these children, but it was for migraine [9]. Both of these studies demonstrated an increasing frequency of TTH in girls over boys during adolescence. As this is also seen in migraine, there remains the possibility of an overlapping evolution of the diagnosis from migraine to TTH and vice versa.

The epidemiological identification of TTH, however, is hampered by the lack of attention paid to these headache disorders, especially when infrequent. Therefore, population-based epidemiology studies may underestimate the prevalence of TTH due to a recall bias, while the inaccuracies of the recall of individual features may overestimate the TTH that should actually be considered migraine. Regardless of these limitations, both migraine and TTH are common pain problems for both children and adults.

10.3 Treatment

Once it has been determined that a patient has TTH, a management plan needs to be developed. As is the case for most headache treatment studies in children, no large-scale treatment studies have been performed with a focus on TTH in children. For adults, several large studies that meet standard study guidelines have been performed (reviewed by Fumal and Schoenen [10]) and the same basic principles of migraine management can be applied to TTH management – acute therapy, preventative therapy and biobehavioral therapy with psychological intervention (for migraine Chapter 8).

Acute therapy

Episodic TTH may be self-limited and may be managed with simple analgesics, such as acetaminophen, and nonsteroidal anti-inflammatory medications (ibuprofen or naproxen sodium). Both of these groups of medicines have been demonstrated to be effective in migraine in children and, by implication, may also be useful in TTH in children.

In addition, as TTH may be mild, but become frequent, the patient and family should be cautioned about the overuse of acute medication and subsequent medication overuse. This may be a major contributor to chronic daily headache. Since a mild TTH with no disability is often treated at home without or with limited medical professional intervention, this needs to be addressed at the initial use of acute medication.

When these simple analgesics are ineffective, a review of the diagnosis should be made and a consideration of migraine or other primary headache treatment initiated. This can include the triptans or indomethacin and may unmask an indomethacin-responsive primary headache.

Preventative therapy

When the TTHs become frequent, preventative therapies may become necessary, especially if disability occurs. This is often the trigger for parents to seek medical attention for their child. For adults, amitriptyline has been demonstrated to be useful for prophylaxis of chronic TTH [11, 12]. The preventative treatment of TTH, however, is lacking and often gets overlapped with the treatment of chronic migraine or chronic daily headache. In adults with chronic TTH, the combination of amitriptyline and cognitive therapy may be even more effective than either one by itself.

Biobehavioral therapy

Biobehavioral therapy includes adherence therapy, lifestyle adjustments and specific psychological interventions, including biofeedback-assisted relaxation therapy [13] and cognitive-behavioral therapy. In a school-based study for the treatment of childhood headaches including TTH, adolescents responded well to relaxation therapies [14]. In children with TTH, biobehavioral therapy has been demonstrated to have prolonged effects over 3 years [15] and may be comparable to amitriptyline [16].

Overall, the treatment plan needs to incorporate all three components to be successful. With time, the TTH may also evolve into migraine or other primary headache disorders and the treatment plan further adjusted [17].

References

1. Headache Classification Subcommittee of the International Headache Society (2004) The International Classification of Headache Disorders. *Cephalagia*, **24**(Suppl. 1), 1–160.

2. Cady, R., Schreiber, C., Farmer, K. and Sheftell, F. (2002) Primary headaches: a convergence hypothesis. *Headache*, **42**, 204–216.

3. Lipton, R.B., Stewart, W.F., Cady, R. *et al.* (2000) Sumatriptan for the range of headaches in migraine sufferers: results of the Spectrum Study. *Headache*, **40**, 783–791.

4. Anttila, P., (2006) Tension-type headache in childhood and adolescence. *Lancet Neurology*, **5**(3), 268–274.

5. Abu-Arafeh, I. and Russell, G. (1994) Prevalence of headache and migraine in school-children. *British Medical Journal*, **309**, 765–769.

6. Barea, J.M., Tannhauser, M. and Rotta, N.T. (1996) An epidemiologic study of headache among children and adolescents of southern Brazil. *Cephalalgia: An International Journal of Headache*, **16**, 545–549.

7. Laurell, K., Larsson, B. and Eeg-Olofsson, O. (2004) Prevalence of headache in Swedish schoolchildren, with a focus on tension-type headache. *Cephalalgia: An International Journal of Headache*, **24**(5), 380–388.

8. Anttila, P., Metsahonkala, L., Aromaa, M. *et al.* (2002) Determinants of tension-type headache in children. *Cephalalgia: An International Journal of Headache*, **22**(5), 401–408.

9. Anttila, P., Metsahonkala, L., Mikkelsson, M. *et al.* (2002) Muscle tenderness in pericranial and neck–shoulder region in children with headache. A controlled study. *Cephalalgia: An International Journal of Headache*, **22**(5), 340–344.

10. Fumal, A. and Schoenen, J. (2008) Tension-type headache: current research and clinical management. *Lancet Neurology*, **7**(1), 70–83.

11. Bedsten, L., Jensen, R. and Olesen, J. (1996) A non-selective (amitriptyline), but not a selective (citalopram), serotonin reuptake inhibitor is effective in the prophylactic treatment of chronic tension-type headache. *Journal of Neurology, Neurosurgery, and Psychiatry*, **61**, 285–290.

12. Gobel, H., Hamouz, V., Hansen, C. *et al.* (1994) Chronic tension-type headache: amitriptyline reduces clinical headache-duration and experimental pain sensitivity but does not alter pericranial muscle activity readings. *Pain*, **59**, 241–249.

13. Bussone, G., Grazzi, L., D'Amico, D. *et al.* (1998) Biofeedback-assisted relaxation training for young adolescents with tension-type headache: a controlled study. *Cephalalgia: An International Journal of Headache*, **18**, 463–467.

14. Larsson, B., Carlsson, J., Fichtel, A. and Melin, L. (2005) Relaxation treatment of adolescent headache sufferers: results from a school-based replication series. *Headache*, **45**(6), 692–704.

15. Grazzi, L., Andrasik, F., D'Amico, D. *et al.* (2001) Electromyographic biofeedback-assisted relaxation training in juvenile episodic tension-type headache: clinical outcome at three-year follow-up. *Cephalalgia: An International Journal of Headache*, **21**(8), 798–803.

16. Grazzi, L., Andrasik, F., Usai, S. *et al.* (2004) Pharmacological behavioural treatment for children and adolescents with tension-type headache: preliminary data. *Neurological Sciences*, **25**(Suppl. 3), S270–S271.

17. Kienbacher, C., Wober, C., Zesch, H.E. *et al.* (2006) Clinical features, classification and prognosis of migraine and tension-type headache in children and adolescents: a long-term follow-up study. *Cephalalgia: An International Journal of Headache*, **26**(7), 820–830.

11

Chronic daily headaches in children

Paul Winner

Children who present with daily, or near-daily, headache represent one of the most challenging subsets of headache. Children with chronic daily headache (CDH) experience significant disability, especially school absences, are often refractory to typical treatment measures and are at risk of overusing over-the-counter (OTC) pain medication.

CDH is formally defined as occurring when there are more than 3 months during which the patient has more than 15 headaches per month that last more than 4 h per day. The majority of teenagers with CDH will report daily headache. The estimated prevalence of CDH is about 1% among adolescents, but it may be as high as 4% in the adult population [1–4]. CDH is a common patient subset in headache clinics, where up to 15 to 30% of patients present with daily or near-daily headache [5].

The quality of life of patients with CDH is often significantly influenced by the pain and associated symptoms [6, 7]. The negative impact extends beyond the affected patient to the family and their friends, as well as to society as a whole. The extensive disability that results from CDH can be measured by school absences, abstinence from after-school activities and the family activities that are disrupted. The parents and teachers are often distraught by the amount of school their children have missed. The parents and the child are often fearful that there is some undiagnosed life-threatening process, a brain tumor for example. It is critical to consider and to exclude possible secondary causes of the headache. No treatment regimen will be successful

Pediatric Headaches in Clinical Practice   Andrew D. Hershey, Paul Winner, Marielle A. Kabbouche and Scott W. Powers
© 2009 John Wiley & Sons, Ltd.

until clear and confident reassurances as to the absence of serious underlying disease are provided.

Early diagnosis and management of CDH is essential and can greatly aid the patient's and family's life and potential to reverse the cycle of disability.

This chapter will describe CDH as it appears in children and to provide management options.

11.1 Classification

The International Classification of Headache Disorders, second edition (ICHD-II) [8], divides headaches into many categories, but the principle separation is between primary headache disorders and secondary headache disorders A chronic daily pattern of headache may be either primary or secondary. This chapter focuses on primary forms of CDH (Table 11.1), but will guide the reader on the appropriate steps to exclude secondary headache etiologies.

The predominant form seen in children at tertiary care clinics is CMs. CMs evolve from an episodic migraine pattern.

Previously referred to as transformed migraine, the term CM has become the more accepted term recently [12, 13]. The differences between this concept of transformation and the ICHD-II criteria have been debated and tested, but some controversy remains [14–16]. The issues are due to the observation that, as migraines become more frequent, there is some loss of migraine features [15, 17]. In an attempt to address this issue, a recommendation by the ICHD-II criteria committee has suggested the use of the appendix in which only 8 days per month require the headache to be migraine with a total frequency of greater than 15 days per month [18]. Although this may still be limiting in the inclusiveness of CM, it does assist with the recognition.

Just as CM evolves from episodic migraine, CTTHs appear to evolve from episodic tension-type headaches. CTTH is considered to be more common than we appreciate because these children may not be brought to a physician's attention because of the lower degrees of disability; this remains to be proven.

Table 11.1 Four categories of primary chronic headache

1. Chronic (transformed) migraine (CM)
2. Chronic tension-type headache (CTTH)
3. New daily persistent headache (NDPH)
4. Hemicranium continuum

The NDPH appears to be a form of CDH that starts quite abruptly, without any history of a previous headache syndrome. The patient can frequently recall the date and even the time then the headache began.

The NDPH pattern has also been noted in children in which an underlying triggering phenomenon, such as infection or minor head trauma, has been identified. When this history is obtained, NDPH could be thought of as a form of secondary headache [9].

Hemicranium continuum, rare in children, represents a cluster variant (trigeminal autonomic cephalalgia) with daily or continuous unilateral pain with conjunctival injection, lacrimation, rhinorrhea and, occasionally, ptosis. One of the most striking features of hemicranium continuum is its responsiveness to indomethacin.

CDH in adult headache clinics breaks down to 78% of the patients were found to have CM and 15.3% were found to have CTTH, whereas NDPH and hemicranium continuum, combined, occurred in 6.7% of patients.

Each of these four types of CDH can be further divided into those with or without medication overuse. The medications implicated in this analgesic overuse syndrome include most OTC analgesics, opioids, butalbital-containing compounds, ergotamine and triptans [10, 11].

The influence of medication overuse has also been noted to be controversial, and the application of the criteria for CM and medication overuse headache (MOH) were felt to be in conflict. This was due to the requirement that the diagnosis of MOH be made after a response to medication cessation was observed. A recommendation not requiring this feature to make the diagnosis of MOH in the presence of CM classification, a suggested modification to the CDH diagnosis [18].

11.2 Epidemiology

The characterization of CDH in children is incomplete; the present discussions relies on the adult experience. Historically, Gladstein and Holden [19] identified a cohort of children with CDH that included patients with intermittent migraine and underlying CTTHs: comorbid headaches (40%), NDPHs (35%) and transformed migraines (15%). They identified a subgroup they termed comorbid headaches in children who had multiple or mixed headache disorders contributing to their CDH. Their follow-up studies, however, did not validate the comorbid subgroup and, in fact, indicated that the majority (64%) of childhood CDHs were migraines or migrainous [20].

Hershey *et al.* [17] assessed a group of 200 children who presented to a tertiary headache center and who had experienced more than 15 headache days per month for at least 3 months, finding that 92% of these children had characteristics suggestive of CM. The frequency of headache was the most significant factor limiting the diagnosis, because 19.5% of the patients had continuous headaches. Three headache subgroups emerged: (1) frequent but not daily headaches, (2) daily intermittent headaches and (3) daily continuous headaches. The patients with headaches that were frequent but not daily had 15 to 29 headache days per month (i.e. at least one headache-free day per month), and their headache features most closely resembled the International Headache Society (IHS) criteria for migraines. The patients with daily intermittent headaches had a headache every day but also had headache-free periods; the features of this subgroup's headaches also aligned most closely with the IHS criteria for migraines. The group with daily continuous headache had headaches with many migrainous features, although there was overlap with the features of tension-type headaches. Both of the above-mentioned studies point to the prominent migrainous nature of headaches in children with CDH.

Seshia [21], in a study of Canadian children referred to a tertiary neurology clinic, found that 31% had CDH; this study continued to demonstrate the difficulty with separating migraine and tension-type headaches when the headaches are frequent with 27% having both headache types.

More information is needed to fully characterize CDH in children.

It is important to exclude secondary causes of CDH in children, such as neoplasms, idiopathic intracranial hypertension, hydrocephalus, chronic subdural hematomas, chronic sinusitis, glaucoma, malocclusion, temporomandibular joint dysfunction and psychological conditions, before you determine your diagnosis.

11.3 Clinical characteristics

Children with CDH will often complain of at least two types of headache [4]. The most prominent are severe intermittent headaches that are migraine in character. The headaches will be described as bifrontal, throbbing, severe, crushing. They are often associated with nausea during the most severe times, and the patient will frequently have photophobia, phonophobia and osmophobia. For this more severe headache pain, sleep will sometimes help, but they will still have persistent headache when they awaken. The frequency of these severe headaches will vary with the individual. The severe episodes typically occur multiple times a week.

In addition to these severe intermittent headaches, the child with CDH will often complain of a continuous or baseline headache that is present 24/7. This continuous headache may wax and wane, often being worse either in the morning or at the end of the school day. The characteristics of the continuous or baseline headache pain are similar to the episodes of severe headaches, only less intense.

In one study looking at 178 patients with CDH, the baseline headache occurred 27.3 ± 4.1 days per month with a mean pain intensity of 5.9 ± 2.1 on a 10-point scale. The superimposed episodic headache occurred 4.7 ± 3.8 days per month with a mean pain intensity of 8.4 ± 1.4 and was more often associated with migrainous symptoms. After logistic regression to control for pain intensity, the only statistically significant difference between the two headache types was a lower prevalence of pain in the superimposed headache. This suggests that, rather than having two coexistent headache types, children with CDH have a syndrome that periodically worsens and demonstrates more severe migrainous symptoms [4].

The occasional patient with CDH may have allodynia over all or part of their head. Allodynia is a sensitivity to touch on part of the scalp or face that may occur with severe headaches. A small percentage of patients may have idiopathic stabbing headaches (ice-pick headaches), which are severe, intermittent, stabbing-like head pains that are often times multifocal, occurring for seconds at a time and happening many times during the day.

Headache is not the only symptom in CDH. Comorbid symptoms include dizziness, sleep disturbance, pain at other sites of the body (including neck pain, back pain and abdominal pain), fatigue, difficulty in concentration, sad mood and increased anxiety. It is important to recognize and treat these other symptoms and avoid medications that could exacerbate these comorbid conditions.

Many CDH patients have symptoms of dizziness. The dizziness is associated with feeling weak and unsteady, and with changes in (blurring or loss of) vision. The dizziness is often positional, and patients will complain of syncope or near syncope several minutes after standing. There is typically no vertigo.

The dizziness is particularly prominent in the morning after they first get up.

During the office examination, a difference in blood pressure or pulse rate between sitting and standing may be noted. The patient often experiences mild symptoms of this dizziness if stood up for several minutes in the office. One may see either a significant tachycardia with standing (postural orthostatic tachycardia syndrome) and/or a decrease in the systolic blood pressure with standing (neurocardiogenic syncope). A tilt-table test will help confirm these impressions.

11.4 Diagnosis

One of the roles of a treating physician for these patients is to distinguish CDH, which is a primary headache syndrome, from other secondary causes of headache and to provide appropriate reassurance to the patients and their family. The evaluation of the young person with CDH will include a thorough history and physical examination, as well as consideration of a neuroimaging study, blood tests and, in the occasional patient, lumbar puncture.

In selected patients, tilt-table testing or sleep studies may also be needed.

The physical examination of children with chronic headache is important; abnormal findings need to explained. Head circumference may disclose macrocrania, a clue toward unrecognized chronic hydrocephalus or subdural collections. The skin examination looks for hints of either neurofibromatosis or tuberous sclerosis.

A fundoscopic examination is necessary to rule out the presence of papilledema and increased intracranial pressure.

Neurologic examination should evaluate the possible presence of focal deficits. Examination of the spine is also done because of the frequent presence of neck and back pain.

Perhaps the most useful role of the neuroimaging study in CDH is to reassure the patient and family [10]. An imaging study is most likely to be significantly abnormal if there are focal deficits on examination or a history of seizures in the patient [11]. Occasionally, incidental vascular anomalies, white-matter abnormalities, arachnoid cysts or pineal cysts will be seen that are generally believed to be of little to no clinical significance in children with CDH but can cause great anxiety for families [12]. If a patient has had a significant history of head or neck trauma, particularly at the onset of the CDH, then magnetic resonance angiography of the neck should also be considered to rule out a possible carotid dissection. When idiopathic intracranial hypertension (IIH) is a strong consideration, then magnetic resonance venography may also be considered since sinus thrombosis can cause elevated intracranial pressure.

Informative serum studies include evaluation of the thyroid. Sedimentation rates could be used to look for evidence of inflammation or an arteritis.

If there are other clinical signs of systemic lupus erythematosus in addition to the headache, then an antinuclear antibodies, erythrocyte sedimentation rate, and C-reactive protein should be obtained.

Many patients will transition from a headache-free period or episodic migraines to CMs during an infection. Consideration should be given to titers for Epstein–Barr virus, West Nile virus and Lyme disease. Although there is no specific treatment for some of the viral etiologies, many of the parents appreciate knowing that there was a physiological etiology for the transition to a chronic headache.

IIH is a constellation of symptoms and signs that include an elevated intracranial pressure with a normal MRI scan. The patient with IIH will complain of a headache, diplopia, tinnitus and eye pain. On examination, the patient will have papilledema and a sixth nerve palsy. Although the diagnosis is easy to make when all these signs and symptoms are present, there are some rare patients who may have IIH without showing significant papilledema.

Rare in children, chronic meningitis due to tuberculosis, fungi or Lyme disease can be present with CDH and a clinical pattern nearly identical to IIH.

Physical examination will demonstrate signs of increased intracranial pressure but imaging studies may prove to be unrevealing. Lumbar puncture with special attention to opening pressure in the lateral recumbent position and specific spinal fluid studies will be necessary.

Patients with CDH or migraine seem to be prone to getting a post-lumbar puncture headache or low-pressure headache. Lumbar puncture can be a valuable diagnostic tool, but one should be cautious about its use because one can make a child's headache significantly worse. When measuring the pressure, effort should be made to minimize the child's anxiety as much possible and the pressure should be measured with the legs extended and the head relaxed.

11.5 Management

The basic principles of management of the adolescent with CDH include identifying and treating the components of the headache syndrome, removing drugs that lead to rebound, assessing prognosis and affording realistic expectations to the family.

The initiation of a multidisciplined approach with emphasis on preventive strategies takes precedence over the use of intermittent analgesics [22, 23]. A comprehensive approach incorporates healthy brain principles, such as regulation of sleep and eating habits, regular exercise, identification of triggering

Table 11.2 Strategies for preventing CDH

Preventive therapies	Biobehavioral therapies
Regular sleep schedule	Stress management
Daily exercise	Vitamins: riboflavin
Dietary measures	Minerals: magnesium
Caffeine avoidance	Herbal supplements: Petadolex (Butter root)
Regular meal schedule	

factors and stress management, as well as biofeedback-assisted relaxation therapy and high-quality supplements and, when necessary, psychological or psychiatric intervention (Table 11.2) [24, 25].

A thorough social and educational history is recommended to explore the potential issues relating to life at school (e.g. bullying, learning disabilities), family conflict (parental discord or impending divorce), grief and drug and alcohol use.

Sleep is frequently disrupted in patients who have CDH [15]. A common sleep disturbance is a delayed onset in sleep, and oftentimes these individuals will not be able to fall asleep for 30 min to several hours after they go to bed. Many children will wake frequently during the night as well. Occasionally, there is a history of pain and restless legs during the night. Consideration can be given to a formal sleep study to evaluate these symptoms. The lack of sleep can be a strong contributing factor that will aggravate the headache symptoms. Typically, the headache syndrome will not resolve until the sleep is improved.

For the CDH population, a group of lifestyle changes must be incorporated into the treatment plan. This is essentially maintenance of a healthy lifestyle and includes four major components: adequate and regular sleep; regular exercise (20 to 30 min of aerobic exercise per day); balanced nutrition (including not skipping meals)/supplements; adequate fluid intake; and moderation of caffeine intake.

The pharmacologic treatment of CDH requires an individualized regimen and the judicious use of appropriate acute and preventative strategies. Recognizing the degree of disability will help guide the management.

11.6 Preventative therapy

The majority of CDH in children is CM; therefore, a modification of standard migraine therapy is appropriate, but the emphasis must be placed on

Table 11.3 Pharmacologic therapies

Antidepressant agents	amitriptyline, 1.0 mg/kg (20–100 mg) orally at bedtime
Antiepileptic agents	topiramate, 25–100 mg orally bid
	valproic acid, 250–500 mg orally bid
Nonsteroidal anti-inflammatory agents	naproxen, 250–500 mg orally bid
Antihypertensive agents	propranolol, 60–120 mg orally once per day
Antihistamines	cyproheptadine, 2–8 mg orally, divided bid or at bedtime

preventative measures. Presently, there is not a single Food and Drug Administration (FDA)-approved preventative medication for use in children, but there is growing support for their use [26].

For patients who have had a recent onset of CDH attributed almost exclusively to analgesic rebound, an analgesic-free period may be all that is necessary for the successful treatment of the child.

Preventative therapies for CDH include the medications that are used in adults, but the dosages and adverse events need to be addressed. Tricyclic antidepressants, antiepileptic agents, beta-blockers, calcium channel blockers and other adult treatments have been and are utilized in the pediatric population (Table 11.3). Few of these medications have been subjected to controlled trials. When making the clinical decision in regard to pharmacologic agents, it is important to consider comorbid conditions. For the patient with difficulty falling asleep, amitriptyline at bedtime may provide added benefits. Similarly, if there are mild to moderate affective issues, then amitriptyline or valproic acid may be beneficial. If there is comorbid obesity, then topiramate may decrease the appetite.

Antidepressants

The tricyclic antidepressant amitriptyline has been widely used as a preventative agent for migraine headaches. Tricyclic antidepressants are tolerated in children; the side effects are attributable to anticholinergic effects, and there are additional concerns about cardiac arrhythmias. The most frequently cited side effects include sedation.

To help minimize side effects, the medicine should be introduced slowly. Starting at 0.25 mg/kg (5–10 mg) and increasing by 0.25 mg every 2 to 3 weeks to a dose of 1.0 mg/kg (10–25 mg) will often result in effective management [27]. Serotonin-specific reuptake inhibitors have not been studied for CDH, but they may have a role for patients with comorbid depression.

Antiepileptic medications

Several antiepileptic drugs have been shown to be approved by the FDA for use as an effective preventative medication in the treatment of adult migraine; they include topiramate and divalproate [28]. Limited evidence on their effect in children is available.

Topiramate, one of the newer antiepileptic drugs, has demonstrated efficacy in preventing adult and adolescent migraine. This multicenter double-blind placebo-controlled multi-dose trial included patients aged 12 to 65 years with a 6-month history of IHS-defined migraine and 3 to 12 migraines per month but excluded patients who experienced more than 15 headache days per month [29]. A significant reduction in headache frequency was demonstrated with doses of 50 to 100 mg twice daily (bid). Adverse events resulting in discontinuation in the topiramate groups included paresthesia, fatigue and nausea.

One retrospective study assessing the efficacy of topiramate for pediatric headache included 41 patients. Daily topiramate doses of 1.4 ± 0.74 mg/kg per day were reached and headache frequency was reduced from 16.5 ± 10 headaches per month to 11.6 ± 10 headaches per month ($p < 0.001$). Mean headache severity, duration and accompanying disability were also reduced. Side effects included cognitive changes (12.5%), weight loss (5.6%) and sensory symptoms (2.8%) [30]. This study population consisted predominantly of children who had very frequent migraine headaches approaching the spectrum of CDH (defined as 15 or more headaches per month).

In the study of CM, both a small study in adults [31] and in children [32], the adult study was a placebo-controlled study that was effective, while the pediatric study was open label, retrospective and only low doses were examined.

Further studies in CM and treatment with topiramate are needed to expand these observations.

The most commonly observed side effects include paresthesias, weight loss, and cognitive problems. The cognitive problems appear to decline with use and can be minimized by a very slow taper starting at a very low dose. This starting dose may be as low as 12.5 mg per day and may be slowly increased by 12.5 mg every 2 weeks to a dose of 50 mg bid [30]. The weight loss needs to be monitored, although it does not appear to be significant for the majority of children.

Divalproate has been shown to be effective and has been approved as a preventative treatment for migraines in adults [33]. It has also been shown to be effective for CDH in an extended-release formulation [34, 35]. A small study with 42 patients demonstrated that it was effective and well tolerated in 7- to 16-year-old patients [36]. Two side effects that may limit its use in adolescents are weight gain and ovarian cysts.

Gabapentin has also been used for prevention of adult headaches. It appears to be well tolerated and effective, but its effectiveness in children remains to be demonstrated [37].

Antihistamines

The antihistamine cyproheptadine has been widely used as a preventative treatment for migraine headaches in young children, but it has not been studied for CDH [38, 39]. It tends to be well tolerated; its most significant side effects are sedation and weight gain.

Beta-blockers

Both propranolol and atenolol are often used as effective preventative agents for migraine in adults. There is conflicting data regarding the efficacy of propranolol for migraine treatment in children [26, 39–41], and there are no data on its use for CDH. The exact dosing parameters also have not been identified. Two of its more common side effects that are of concern for children are exacerbation of reactive airway disease and depression. This reactive airway disease may be of special concern for the athletic children, who are unaware of it until the combination of exercise and a beta-blocker results in shortness of breath.

Nonsteroidal anti-inflammatory drugs

Naproxen sodium, a nonsteroidal anti-inflammatory drug (NSAID), was shown to be an effective treatment for adolescent migraine in one small ($n = 10$) trial with a double-blind placebo-controlled crossover design [26]. Sixty percent of the patients experienced a reduction of 60% in headache frequency and severity with naproxen (250 mg bid), whereas only 40% responded favorably to placebo. No severe adverse effects were reported in this study. Naproxen should not be used for longer than 8 weeks because of potential gastrointestinal toxicity in this population without proper supervision.

11.7 Analgesic agents

Medication overuse may be one of the precipitants of CDH, so care must be taken not to contribute to the overuse of analgesic agents. For effective analgesia the child and parents need to treat the migraine early, using an adequate dose and avoiding overuse. Avoid using analgesic medication more than three times per week.

Catching the migraine headache component at the onset may be difficult in children with CDH because some children experience a rapid worsening of their headaches. Some children have a strong ability to distract themselves and may not detect the headache until it is severe or until vomiting occurs. For analgesic therapies in general, the earlier the treatment, the more effective it will be; hence, the need to emphasize to children and the parent the importance of early recognition and intervention.

The second important key to effective analgesic use is proper dosing.

For ibuprofen, the effective dose appears to be 10 mg/kg, although some studies have used a 7.5 mg/kg dose for effective management of migraine headaches [42, 43]. Underdosing runs the risk of headache recurrence and rebound that may be more difficult to treat and that may progress to analgesic rebound. MOH is a well-recognized headache phenomenon where by the overuse of acute medications increases headache frequency. Analgesic overuse has been proposed as one of the prime causes of transformed migraines in both adults and children [4, 44].

The third component of analgesic therapy is limiting its use. A typical limitation for an abortive treatment is to use it no more than two to three times per week; this also includes migraine-specific medications. This is done to prevent the development analgesic rebound headaches.

Limiting the use of analgesics to two to three times per week may be exceptionally difficult for the CDH sufferers who are having headaches nearly every day. Some patients are able to identify a spectrum of severity and can, therefore, use their acute therapy for the most severe two to three headaches per week [45, 46]. Many children are unable to identify the episodes of migraine within their pattern of CDH until the headache has reached peak severity.

The addition of a sliding-scale treatment approach has been employed for the acute treatment of episodic migraine [47]. In this model, an NSAID is used for mild to moderate severity, while a combination of an NSAID and a triptan is used for moderate to severe headaches.

The application of this model with strict limitations on the frequency of use may assist those children with CM that have an occasional severe headache.

Analgesic withdrawal

The subset of children overusing analgesics poses a particularly difficult challenge, because they must be taken off these agents before any other regimen can be implemented. When it is necessary to stop an offending acute agent, several approaches may be used alone or in combination.

Dihydroergotamine is effective for status migrainous, and some patients will get pain relief for their chronic pain [17]. Valproate also comes in an intravenous (IV) formulation and has been used to abort severe headache episodes [18]. Some children respond to a short-term use of oral steroids or IV steroids [19]. Some children with chronic headache symptoms will need to be hospitalized for these treatments but are at risk of reverting to their typical headache after leaving the hospital. The hospitalization may provide the child an opportunity for education about headaches, introduction to biofeedback and in some cases physical therapy. It also gives the physician a window into the family dynamics often not assessable in the busy office setting.

11.8 Nonpharmacologic

A variety of vitamins (e.g. riboflavin [48], coenzyme Q10 [49]), minerals (e.g. magnesium) [50] and herbal remedies (e.g. feverfew [51], butterbur [52, 53]) have been used for prevention of adult headaches. Unfortunately, most of these have not been evaluated in children, nor have they been clearly evaluated for CDH, but they may play a beneficial role, particularly for families for which traditional pharmacologic approaches are less effective or unacceptable.

Biofeedback-assisted relaxation therapy has been shown to be effective in aborting and preventing recurrent headaches in children. This technique is typically taught through multisession analysis. It can also be effectively taught in a single session with a tape provided for practicing at home [54]. It requires a degree of motivation in the child, and it is difficult to assess its effectiveness in isolation. It has a low potential for side effects. A combination approach of nonpharmacologic and pharmacologic treatments tends to be the most effective management.

Psychiatric intervention

The multidisciplinary approach with biobehavioral management of CDH is an essential part of the treatment plan and includes a balancing of lifestyle habits and adherence to the treatment regimen [55]. This may be complicated by comorbid psychological conditions that require further interventions.

In adults, an association between migraine/CDH and depression has been demonstrated [56]. In addition, stress has been implicated as a possible migraine trigger. Psychological/psychiatric intervention for identifying these possible components may be essential in the management of CDH.

11.9 Prognosis

Limited long-term follow-up data exist for the population of children and adolescents with CDH. Lewis *et al.* [57] reported a short-term (6 months) follow-up on 39 adolescents, peak age 13 years, with CDH of whom greater than half experienced a ≥75% reduction in headache frequency and one-third a ≥90% improvement in a 6-month follow-up. A wide variety of preventive agents were employed, but amitriptyline, amitriptyline plus naproxen, and topiramate provided the largest proportion of successful outcomes [57]. Further research is needed.

11.10 Conclusions

CDH in children can be a challenging form of primary headache to manage. The first step is to establish the diagnosis and to provide the necessary reassurances to the family that there is no life-threatening illness. The next step is to eliminate aggravating or exacerbating phenomena, such as analgesic or caffeine overuse, and to create a comprehensive management program that incorporates bio-behavioral measures, lifestyle modifications along with the daily preventive medicines, and the judicious and limited use of analgesics. The choice of daily medicines should be based upon exploration of comorbid conditions, such as sleep disturbances or emotional considerations.

Realistic expectations for the treatment of CDH need to be clearly outlined to both the child and the parents. It is difficult for many families to comprehend that the headaches can persist for such a long time that there are no abnorm-alities showing up on diagnostic testing and that the medications they are prescribed are not immediately effective. It is not unusual for patients with chronic headache to see multiple doctors. It is important to spend adequate time discussing the nature of CDH, how secondary causes of headache have been ruled out, the role of medications, how to avoid OTC pain relievers, the role of biofeedback or physical therapy, and stress that a comprehensive approach is necessary.

References

1. Abu-Arafeh, I. and Russell, G. (1994) Prevalence of headache and migraine in school children. *British Medical Journal*, **309**, 765–769.
2. Lipton, R.B. and Stewart, W.F. (1997) Prevalence and impact of migraine. *Neurologic Clinics*, **15**, 1–13.
3. Castillo, J., Munoz, P., Guitera, V. and Pascual, J. (1999) Epidemiology of chronic daily headache in the general population. *Headache*, **39**, 190–196.
4. Wang, S.J., Fuh, J.L., Lu, S.R. and Juang, K.D. (2006) Chronic daily headache in adolescents: prevalence, impact, and medication overuse. *Neurology*, **66**(2), 193–197.
5. Viswanathan, V., Bridges, S.J., Whitehouse, W. and Newton, R.W. (1998) Childhood headaches: discrete entities or continuum? *Developmental Medicine and Child Neurology*, **40**(8), 544–550.
6. Powers, S.W., Patton, S.R., Hommel, K.A. and Hershey, A.D. (2003) Quality of life in childhood migraines: clinical impact and comparison to other chronic illnesses. *Pediatrics*, **112**(1), (Pt 1), e1–e5.
7. Guitera, V., Munoz, P., Castillo, J. and Pascual, J. (2002) Quality of life in chronic daily headache. *Neurology*, **58**, 1062–1065.
8. Headache Classification Subcommittee of the International Headache (2004) The International Classification of Headache Disorders. *Cephalalgia: An International Journal of Headache*, **24**(Suppl 1), 1–160.
9. Mack, K.J. (2004) What incites new daily persistent headache in children? *Pediatric Neurology*, **31**(2), 122–125.
10. Mathew, N.T., Kurman, R. and Perez, F. (1990) Drug induced refractory headache – clinical features and management. *Headache*, **30**, 633–637.
11. Meskunas, C.A., Tepper, S.J., Rapoport, A.M. *et al.* (2006) Medications associated with probable medication overuse headache reported in a tertiary care headache center over a 15-year period. *Headache*, **46**(5), 766–772.
12. Guitera, V., Munoz, P., Castillo, J. and Pascual, J. (1999) Transformed migraine: a proposal for the modification of its diagnostic criteria based on recent epidemiological data. *Cephalalgia: An International Journal of Headache*, **19**, 847–850.
13. Silberstein, S. and Lipton, R. (2001) Chronic daily headache including transformed migraine, chronic tension-type headache, and medication over-use, in Wolff's Headache and Other Head Pain, 7th edn (eds S.D. Silberstein, R.B. Lipton and D.J. Dalessio), Oxford University Press, New York, pp. 247–282.
14. Bigal, M.E., Tepper, S.J., Sheftell, F.D. *et al.* (2004) Chronic daily headache: correlation between the 2004 and the 1988 International Headache Society diagnostic criteria. *Headache*, **44**(7), 684–691.
15. Bigal, M.E., Rapoport, A.M., Tepper, S.J. *et al.* (2005) The classification of chronic daily headache in adolescents – a comparison between the second edition of the international classification of headache disorders and alternative diagnostic criteria. *Headache*, **45**(5), 582–589.
16. Bigal, M.E., Tepper, S.J., Sheftell, F.D. *et al.* (2006) Field testing alternative criteria for chronic migraine. *Cephalalgia: An International Journal of Headache*, **26**(4), 477–482.

17. Hershey, A.D., Powers, S.W., Bentti, A.L. *et al.* (2001) Characterization of chronic daily headaches in children in a multidisciplinary headache center. *Neurology,* **56**(8), 1032–1037.

18. Olesen, J., Bousser, M.G., Diener, H.C. *et al.* (2006) New appendix criteria open for a broader concept of chronic migraine. *Cephalalgia: An International Journal of Headache,* **26**(6), 742–746.

19. Gladstein, J. and Holden, E.W. (1996) Chronic daily headache in children and adolescents: a 2-year prospective study. *Headache,* **36**, 349–351.

20. Koenig, M.A., Gladstein, J., McCarter, R.J. *et al.* (2002) Chronic daily headache in children and adolescents presenting to tertiary headache clinics. *Headache,* **42**(6), 491–500.

21. Seshia, S.S. (2004) Chronic daily headache in children and adolescents. *The Canadian Journal of Neurological Sciences,* **31**(3), 319–323.

22. Redillas, C. and Solomon, S. (2000) Prophylactic pharmacological treatment of chronic daily headache. *Headache,* **40**, 83–102.

23. Bigal, M.E. and Lipton, R.B. (2006) The preventive treatment of migraine. *Neurologist,* **12** (4), 204–213.

24. Rothrock, J.F. (1999) Management of chronic daily headache utilizing a uniform treatment pathway. *Headache,* **39**, 650–653.

25. Magnusson, J.E., Becker, W.J. and Riess, C.M., (2004) Effectiveness of a multidisciplinary treatment program for chronic daily headache. *The Canadian Journal of Neurological Sciences,* **31**(1), 72–79.

26. Lewis, D., Ashwal, S., Hershey, A. *et al.* (2004) Practice parameter: pharmacological treatment of migraine headache in children and adolescents: report of the American Academy of Neurology Quality Standards Subcommittee and the Practice Committee of the Child Neurology Society. *Neurology,* **63**(12), 2215–2224.

27. Hershey, A.D., Powers, S.W., Bentti, A.L. and Degrauw, T.J. (2000) Effectiveness of amitriptyline in the prophylactic management of childhood headaches. *Headache,* **40**(7), 539–549.

28. Bartolini, M., Silvestrini, M., Taffi, R. *et al.* (2005) Efficacy of topiramate and valproate in chronic migraine. *Clinical Neuropharmacology,* **28**(6), 277–279.

29. Brandes, J.L., Saper, J.R., Diamond, M. *et al.* (2004) Topiramate for migraine prevention: a randomized controlled trial. *The Journal of the American Medical Association,* **291**(8), 965–973.

30. Hershey, A.D., Powers, S.W., Vockell, A.L. *et al.* (2002) Effectiveness of topiramate in the prevention of childhood headaches. *Headache,* **42**(8), 965–973.

31. Silvestrini, M., Bartolini, M., Coccia, M. *et al.* (2003) Topiramate in the treatment of chronic migraine. *Cephalalgia: An International Journal of Headache,* **23**(8), 820–824.

32. Borzy, J.C., Koch, T.K. and Schimschock, J.R. (2005) Effectiveness of topiramate in the treatment of pediatric chronic daily headache. *Pediatric Neurology,* **33**(5), 314–316.

33. Mathew, N.T., Saper, J.R., Silberstein, S.D. *et al.* (1995) Migraine prophylaxis with divalproex. *Archives of Neurology,* **52**, 281–286.

34. Freitag, F., Diamond, S., Diamond, M.L. and Urban, G.J. (2001) Divalproex in the long-term treatment of chronic daily headache. *Headache,* **41**, 271–278.

35. Freitag, F., Collins, S.D., Carlson, H.A. *et al.* (2002) A randomized trial of divalproex sodium extended-release tablets in migraine prophylaxis. *Neurology*, **58**, 1652–1659.

36. Caruso, J.M., Brown, W.D., Exil, G. and Gascon, G.G. (2000) The efficacy of divalproex sodium in the prophylactic treatment of children with migraine. *Headache*, **40**, 672–676.

37. Mathew, N.T., Rapoport, A., Saper, J. *et al.* (2001) Efficacy of gabapentin in migraine prophylaxis. *Headache*, **41**, 119–128.

38. Bille, B., Ludvigsson, J. and Sanner, G. (1977) Prophylaxis of migraine in children. *Headache*, **17**, 61–63.

39. Levinstein, B. (1991) A comparative study of cyproheptadine, amitriptyline, and propranolol in the treatment of adolescent migraine. *Cephalalgia: An International Journal of Headache*, **11**, 122–123.

40. Ludvigsson, J. (1974) Propranolol used in prophylaxis of migraine in children. *Acta Neurologica Scandinavica*, **50**, 109–115.

41. Ziegler, D.K. and Hurwitz, A. (1993) Propranolol and amitriptyline in prophylaxis of migraine. *Archives of Neurology*, **50**, 825–830.

42. Hämäläinen, M.L., Hoppu, K., Valkeila, E. and Santavuori, P. (1997) Ibuprofen or acetaminophen for the acute treatment of migraine in children. *Neurology*, **48**, 103–107.

43. Lewis, D., Kellstein, D., Dahl, G. *et al.* (2001) Children's ibuprofen suspension for pediatric migraine. *Annals of Neurology*, **50**(3), (Suppl 1), S93.

44. Vasconcellos, E., Pina-Garza, J.E., Millan, E.J. and Warner, J.S. (1998) Analgesic rebound headache in children and adolescents. *Journal of Child Neurology*, **13**(9), 443–447.

45. Lipton, R.B., Stewart, W.F., Cady, R. *et al.* (2000) Sumatriptan for the range of headaches in migraine sufferers: results of the Spectrum Study. *Headache*, **40**, 783–791.

46. Cady, R.C., Ryan, R., Jhingran, P. *et al.* (1998) Sumatriptan injection reduces productivity loss during a migraine attack: results of a double-blind, placebo-controlled trial. *Archives of Internal Medicine*, **9**, 1013–1018.

47. Smith, T.R., Sunshine, A., Stark, S.R. *et al.* (2005) Sumatriptan and naproxen sodium for the acute treatment of migraine. *Headache*, **45**(8), 983–991.

48. Schoenen, J., Jacquy, J. and Lenaerts, M. (1998) Effectiveness of high-dose riboflavin in migraine prophylaxis: a randomized controlled trial. *Neurology*, **50**, 466–470.

49. Sandor, P.S., Di Clemente, L., Coppola, G. *et al.* (2005) Efficacy of coenzyme Q10 in migraine prophylaxis: a randomized controlled trial. *Neurology*, **64**(4), 713–715.

50. Pfaffenrath, V., Wessely, P., Meyer, C. *et al.* (1996) Magnesium in the prophylaxis of migraine – a double-blind, placebo-controlled study. *Cephalalgia: An International Journal of Headache*, **16**, 436–440.

51. Vogler, B.K., Pittler, M.H. and Ernst, E. (1998) Feverfew as a preventive treatment for migraine: a systematic review. *Cephalalgia: An International Journal of Headache*, **18**, 704–708.

52. Lipton, R.B., Gobel, H., Einhaupl, K.M. *et al.* (2004) *Petasites hybridus* root (butterbur) is an effective preventive treatment for migraine. *Neurology*, **63**(12), 2240–2244.

53. Pothmann, R. and Danesch, U. (2005) Migraine prevention in children and adolescents: results of an open study with a special butterbur root extract. *Headache*, **45**(3), 196–203.

54. Powers, S.W. and Hershey, A.D. (2002) Biofeedback for childhood migraine, in Current Management in Child Neurology, 2nd edn (ed. B.L. Maria), B.C. Decker, Hamilton, ON, pp. 83–85.

55. Powers, S.W. and Andrasik, F. (2005) Biobehavioral treatment, disability, and psychological effects of pediatric headache. *Pediatric Annals*, **34**(6), 461–465.

56. Juant, K.-D., Wang, S.-J., Fuh, J.-L. *et al.* (2000) Comorbidity of depressive and anxiety disorders in chronic daily headache and its subtypes. *Headache*, **40**, 818–823.

57. Lewis, D.W., Harvey, H. and Oakley, C. (2004) Outcome of chronic daily headache in children. *Annals of Neurology*, **36**(8), 107–108.

12

Other primary headache disorders

Marielle A. Kabbouche

This chapter reviews rare headaches that are classified by the The International Classification of Headache Disorders, second edition (ICHD-II) criteria as primary headache due to the negative work-up, such as neuroimaging and physical examination.

These headaches are combined under the trigeminal autonomic cephalalgias (TACs) group in the ICHD-II criteria due to prominent associated autonomic syndromes, but they differ in frequency and duration of attack.

These syndromes are more frequent in the adult population but still occur in childhood and adolescence.

Proper diagnosis is crucial, since therapy is very specific and very effective in most of them.

The ICHD-II coding for these syndromes is shown in Table 12.1.

12.1 Introduction

The trigeminal autonomic cephalalgias share the clinical features of headache and prominent cranial parasympathetic autonomic features. Experimental and human functional imaging suggests that these syndromes activate a normal human trigeminal-parasympathetic reflex with clinical signs of cranial sympathetic dysfunction being secondary.

Pediatric Headaches in Clinical Practice   Andrew D. Hershey, Paul Winner, Marielle A. Kabbouche and Scott W. Powers
© 2009 John Wiley & Sons, Ltd.

Table 12.1 ICHD-II coding for cluster headache and other TACs. (ICHD-II criteria reproduced with permission from Blackwell Publishing)

3-CLUSTER HEADACHE AND OTHER TRIGEMINAL AUTONOMIC CEPHALALGIAS

3.1   *Cluster headache*
    3.1.1   Episodic cluster headache
    3.1.2   Chronic cluster headache
3.2   *Paroxysmal hemicrania*
    3.2.1   Episodic paroxysmal hemicrania (EPH)
    3.2.2   Chronic paroxysmal hemicrania (CPH)
3.3   *Short-lasting unilateral neuralgiform headache attacks with conjunctival injection and tearing(SUNCT)*
3.4   *Probable trigeminal autonomic cephalalgia*
    3.4.1   Probable cluster headache
    3.4.2   Probable paroxysmal hemicrania
    3.4.3   Probable SUNCT
Coded elsewhere:
4.7   *Hemicrania continua*

Hemicrania continua was classified under 4- in the ICHD-II due to less constant cranial autonomic features.

During the first evaluation of a typical presenting TAC it is important to evaluate the patient appropriately to rule out any underlying cause and a secondary symptomatology. The main question that needs to be asked at this time is: 'Primary or secondary headache or both?'

When a headache with the characteristics of a TAC occurs for the first time in close temporal relation to another disorder that is a known cause of headache, it is coded according to the causative disorder as a secondary headache. When a pre-existing TAC is made worse in close temporal relation to another disorder that is a known cause of headache, there are two possibilities and judgment is required. The patient can either be given only the TAC diagnosis or can be given both the TAC diagnosis and a secondary headache diagnosis according to the other disorder. Factors that support adding the latter diagnosis are a very close temporal relation to the disorder, a marked worsening of the TAC, very good evidence that the disorder can cause or aggravate the TAC and, finally, improvement or resolution of the TAC after relief from the disorder.

12.2 Cluster headache

Cluster headache is a well-defined disorder that mostly affects male adults, with a male : female ratio of 2.1 : 1–6.7 : 1 [1]. Age at onset is usually 20–40 years. For unknown reasons, prevalence is three to four times higher in men than in women. The prevalence in children aged 11–18 years has shown a prevalence of 0.1%. Cases in children are rare but have been reported. Acute attacks involve activation of the posterior hypothalamic gray matter. Cluster headache may be inherited (autosomal dominant) in about 5% of cases [2–4].

Clinical features

Patients with the disorder describe episodes of cluster of attacks occurring for weeks and separated by months or years of headache-free periods. The cluster of headaches can occur daily up to eight per day. The attacks are brief, lasting from 15 to 180 min and tend to occur at the same time every day. These attacks do cycle every few months to years. The pain is excruciating, tending to awaken patients from sleep. The patient is described as restless in distress roaming the room. It is a unilateral pain, mostly temporal, but does irradiate to the eyes, neck and jaws. The pain is acute and is associated with one or more autonomic symptoms ipsilateral to the pain. These symptoms include ptosis, miosis, lacrimation, conjunctival injection and rhinorrhea. In a large series with a good follow-up, 27% of patients had only a single cluster period. About 10–15% of patients have chronic symptoms without remissions. During a cluster period, and in the chronic subtype, attacks occur regularly and may be provoked by alcohol, histamine or nitroglycerine.

Previously used terms for this headache include: ciliary neuralgia, erythro-melalgia of the head, erythroprosopalgia of Bing, hemicrania angioparalytica, hemicrania neuralgiformis chronica, histaminic cephalalgia, Horton's head-ache, Harris–Horton's disease, migrainous neuralgia (of Harris), petrosal neuralgia (of Gardner), Sluder's neuralgia, spheno-palatine neuralgia, vidian neuralgia.

ICHD-II criteria

The ICHD-II diagnostic criteria for cluster headaches are given in Table 12.2.

Episodic cluster headache versus chronic cluster headache

Episodic cluster headache

Episodic cluster headache attacks occur in periods lasting 7 days to 1 year separated by pain-free periods lasting 1 month or longer.

The diagnostic criteria are given in Table 12.3.

Table 12.2   ICHD-II diagnostic criteria for cluster headaches. (ICHD-II criteria reproduced with permission from Blackwell Publishing)

A.   At least five attacks fulfilling criteria B–D.
B.   Severe or very severe unilateral orbital, supraorbital and/or temporal pain lasting *15–180 min if untreated.*
C.   Headache is accompanied by *at least one* of the following:
    1.   ipsilateral conjunctival injection and/or lacrimation;
    2.   ipsilateral nasal congestion and/or rhinorrhea;
    3.   ipsilateral eyelid edema;
    4.   ipsilateral forehead and facial sweating;
    5.   ipsilateral miosis and/or ptosis;
    6.   a sense of restlessness or agitation.
D.   Attacks have a frequency from *one every other day to eight per day.*
E.   Not attributed to another disorder.

Notes
1.   During part (but less than half) of the time-course of cluster headache, attacks may be less severe and/or of shorter or longer duration.
2.   During part (but less than half) of the time-course of cluster headache, attacks may be less frequent.
3.   History and physical and neurological examinations do not suggest any of the disorders listed in groups 5–12, or history and/or physical and/or neurological examinations do suggest such disorder but it is ruled out by appropriate investigations, or such disorder is present but attacks do not occur for the first time in close temporal relation to the disorder [5].

Comment
Cluster headache with coexistent trigeminal neuralgia (cluster-tic syndrome) [4, 6, 7]: some patients have been described who have both 3.1 *Cluster headache* and 13.1 *Trigeminal neuralgia.* They should receive both diagnoses. The importance of this observation is that both conditions must be treated for the patient to be headache free.

Table 12.3   Diagnostic criteria for episodic cluster headaches

A.   Attacks fulfilling criteria A–E for 3.1 *Cluster headache.*
B.   At least two cluster periods lasting 7–365 days and separated by pain-free remission periods of ≥1 month.

Note
1.   Cluster periods usually last between 2 weeks and 3 months.

The duration of the remission period has been increased in ICHD-II to a minimum of 1 month.

Chronic cluster headache

Chronic cluster headache attacks are those that occur for more than 1 year without remission or with remissions lasting less than 1 month. The diagnostic criteria are given in Table 12.4.

Table 12.4 Diagnostic criteria for chronic cluster headaches

A. Attacks fulfilling criteria A–E for 3.1 *Cluster headache*
B. Attacks recur over >1 year without remission periods or with remission periods lasting <1 month

Chronic cluster headache may arise *de novo* (previously referred to as *primary chronic cluster headache*) or evolve from the episodic subtype (previously referred to as *secondary chronic cluster headache*). Some patients may switch from chronic to episodic cluster headache.

Treatment of cluster headache

Management of acute attacks

Owing to the acuity and severity of the attack, treatment of an acute episode should be rapid and effective. Oral medications will not be an option for the acute treatment, and other medication with rapid onset should be used [8]:

1. Oxygen.Oxygen inhalation is well tolerated. It is given via a nonrebreathing mask at 7–12 L/min for 20 min. Efficacy is 70% and may work in 5–20 min. It is more effective at the maximum intensity of the pain.

2. Triptan.Injectable and nasal forms are used for acute attacks. A response of 74% of treated patients with subcutaneous sumatriptan was noticed in 15 min after use.

3. Topical local anesthetics.Local intranasal anesthetic agents such as lidocaine have been reported. Lidocaine 4–6% nasal drops (1 ml) may be used and repeated once every 15 min. It is mostly used as an adjunct therapy.

Prophylactic treatment

The goal of preventive therapy is not only to prevent attacks, but also to shorten the ictal phase, as well as decreasing the daily frequency and the occurrence of the bouts. Medications that are used as prophylactic treatments include verapamil, lithium and corticosteroids. It has also been suggested that valproic acid, gabapentin and topiramate can be effective in this condition.

Treatment-resistant patients may benefit from a number of different surgical procedures, including: (1) a sphenopalatine ganglionectomy; (2) a trigeminal surgery; (3) gamma knife radiosurgery.

12.3 Paroxysmal hemicrania

Paroxysmal hemicrania and SUNCT are frequently mistaken for cluster headaches. These syndromes differ primarily in their frequency, duration and treatment response.

Clinical features

Attacks have similar characteristics of pain and associated symptoms and signs to those of cluster headache, but they are *shorter lasting, more frequent* and occur more commonly in *females* with a ratio of 2 : 1; there is no male predominance. Onset is usually in adulthood, although childhood cases are reported [9].

These headaches are rare and benign, and a family history of migraine is reported in 21% of diagnosed patients. The headache is unilateral; the maximum pain is felt in the temporal area as well as in the orbital, maxillary and frontal area. The pain may sometime be less crucial than in cluster headache and is described as a throbbing, boring pain that can vary from moderate to excruciating. Patients are less distressed than in cluster headache and prefer a silent, quiet dark room to lie down in than to be pacing around.

The frequency of attacks is higher than in cluster headache, occurring at a rate of 15 or more attacks per day. The frequency is higher in CPH, where attacks can occur from 1 to 40 times a day. The individual headaches last between 2 and 30 min, with a range of 2–120 min (shorter than cluster headache). The cluster lasts up to 2 weeks to 4 months, with an interictal phase from 1 to 36 months. The pain is associated with one or more autonomic features that are ipsilateral to the pain. These autonomic features, as in cluster headache, include ptosis, conjunctival lacrimation and rhinorrhea. In the ICHD first edition, all parox-ysmal hemicranias were referred to as *CPH*. Sufficient clinical evidence for the episodic subtype has accumulated to separate it in a manner analogous to cluster headache.

As in cluster headaches, it is crucial to rule out an underlying pathology prior to giving the diagnosis of primary headache. A prudent work-up is necessary if a patient presents with these features. Disorders that can mimic paroxysmal hemicrania include aneurysms of the circle of Willis, arterio-venous malforma-tions, strokes, Pancoast tumor, cavernous sinus disorders and other intracranial disorders that can affect the trigeminal path [10].

Diagnostic criteria

The diagnostic criteria for paroxysmal hemicrania are given in Table 12.5.

Table 12.5   Diagnostic criteria for paroxysmal hemicrania [11].

A.   At least 20 attacks fulfilling criteria B–D.
B.   Attacks of severe unilateral orbital, supraorbital or temporal pain lasting 2–30 min.
C.   Headache is accompanied by at least one of the following:
    1.   ipsilateral conjunctival injection and/or lacrimation;
    2.   ipsilateral nasal congestion and/or rhinorrhea;
    3.   ipsilateral eyelid edema;
    4.   ipsilateral forehead and facial sweating;
    5.   ipsilateral miosis and/or ptosis.
D.   Attacks have a frequency above five per day for more than half of the time, although periods with lower frequency may occur.
E.   Attacks are prevented completely by therapeutic doses of indomethacin.[1]
F.   Not attributed to another disorder.[2]

Notes
1.   In order to rule out incomplete response, indomethacin should be used in a dose of $\geq$150 mg daily orally or rectally, or $\geq$100 mg by injection; but for maintenance, smaller doses are often sufficient.
2.   History and physical and neurological examinations do not suggest any of the disorders listed in groups 5–12, or history and/or physical and/or neurological examinations do suggest such disorder but it is ruled out by appropriate investigations, or such disorder is present but attacks do not occur for the first time in close temporal relation to the disorder.

Paroxysmal hemicrania with coexistent trigeminal neuralgia (CPH-tic syndrome)
Patients who fulfill criteria for both 3.2 *Paroxysmal hemicrania* and 13.1 *Trigeminal neuralgia* should receive both diagnoses. The importance of this observation is that both conditions require treatment. The pathophysiological significance of the association is not yet clear.

EPH versus CPH

EPH

Attacks of EPH occur in periods lasting 7 days to 1 year separated by pain-free periods lasting ≥1 month. The diagnostic criteria are given in Table 12.6.

Table 12.6 Diagnostic criteria for EPH

A. Attacks fulfilling criteria A–F for 3.2 *Paroxysmal hemicrania.*
B. At least two attack periods lasting 7–365 days and separated by pain-free remission periods of ≥1 month.

CPH

Attacks of CPH occur for >1 year without remission or with remissions lasting <1 month. The diagnostic criteria are given in Table 12.7.

Table 12.7 Diagnostic criteria for CPH

A. Attacks fulfilling criteria A–F for 3.2 *Paroxysmal hemicrania*
B. Attacks recur over >1 year without remission periods or with remission periods lasting <1 month

Treatment of paroxysmal hemicrania

The standard initial treatment of paroxysmal hemicrania is indomethacin. This syndrome is well known to be very sensitive to indomethacin, which differentiates it from other TACs.

The initial dose is 25 mg three times a day, which can be increased gradually after a week to 50 mg three times a day. If the patient is still unresponsive 2 weeks later, then the dose can be pushed up to 75 mg three times a day [12, 13].

12.4 SUNCT: Short-lasting unilateral neuralgiform headache attacks with conjunctival injection and tearing

This form of primary headache is also a rare form of headache that is associated with autonomic syndromes.

This syndrome is characterized by short-lasting attacks of unilateral pain that are much briefer than those seen in any other TAC and very often accompanied by prominent lacrimation and redness of the ipsilateral eye [14–17].

Clinical features

Patients are usually men, with a male : female ratio of 17 : 2. Age of onset ranges from 10 to 77 years. The headache occurs in paroxysms, as in other TACs, but is shorter in duration: 5–250 s. The episodes occur up to 30 times per hour with an average of 5–6 per hour. The conjunctival injection is the most prominent feature in this syndrome; other autonomic symptoms can still be seen.

The pain is unilateral and can be triggered by mechanical movements of the head.

SUNCT can be mimicked by other intracranial pathologies that need to be carefully ruled out before labeling patients with primary headache. The differential diagnosis should include the following: homolateral cerebellopontine arterio-venous malformations, brain stem cavernous angioma and other structural abnormalities in the posterior fossa [18–21].

Diagnostic criteria

The diagnostic criteria for SUNCT are given in Table 12.8.

Table 12.8 Diagnostic criteria for SUNCT

A. At least 20 attacks fulfilling criteria B–D.
B. Attacks of unilateral orbital, supraorbital or temporal stabbing or pulsating pain lasting 5–240 s.
C. Pain is accompanied by ipsilateral conjunctival injection and lacrimation.
D. Attacks occur with a frequency from 3 to 200 per day.
E. Not attributed to another disorder.[1]

Note
1. History and physical and neurological examinations do not suggest any of the disorders listed in groups 5–12, or history and/or physical and/or neurological examinations do suggest such disorder but it is ruled out by appropriate investigations, or such disorder is present but attacks do not occur for the first time in close temporal relation to the disorder.

This syndrome was described after the publication of the first edition of the ICHD and has become well recognized in the last decade. Patients may be seen with only one of either conjunctival injection or tearing, or other cranial autonomic symptoms such as nasal congestion, rhinorrhea or eyelid edema may be seen. 3.3 *SUNCT* may be a subform of A3.3 *Short-lasting Unilateral neuralgiform headache attacks with cranial autonomic symptoms* (SUNA), described in the appendix. The literature suggests that the most common mimics of 3.3 *SUNCT* are lesions in the posterior fossa or involving the pituitary gland.

Patients have been described in whom there is an overlap between 3.3 *SUNCT* and 13.1 *Trigeminal neuralgia* (i.e. *SUNCT with coexistent trigeminal neuralgia*). Such patients should receive both diagnoses. This differentiation is clinically difficult.

Treatment of SUNCT

SUNCT is known as a refractory TAC. Indomethacin is not useful for acute attacks. Sumatriptan has been used with some response. Preventive therapy, such as gabapentin, topiramate and others, can be tried to decrease the frequency of the attacks.

12.5 Probable TAC

Probable TACs are headache attacks that are believed to be a subtype of TAC but which do not quite meet the diagnostic criteria for any of the subtypes described above. The diagnostic criteria for probable TACs are given in Table 12.9.

Table 12.9   Diagnostic criteria for probable TAC

A.   Attacks fulfilling all but one of the specific criteria for one of the subtypes of TAC.
B.   Not attributed to another disorder.

Comment
Patients coded as 3.4 *Probable TAC* or one of its subforms either have had an insufficient number of typical attacks or fail to fulfill one of the other criteria.

Probable cluster headache

The diagnostic criteria for probable cluster headaches are given in Table 12.10.

Table 12.10   Diagnostic criteria for probable cluster headache

---

A.   Attacks fulfilling all but one of criteria A–D for 3.1 *Cluster headache*.
B.   Not attributed to another disorder.

Probable paroxysmal hemicrania

The diagnostic criteria for probable paroxysmal hemicrania are given in Table 12.11.

Table 12.11   Diagnostic criteria for probable paroxysmal hemicrania

A. Attacks fulfilling all but one of criteria A–E for 3.2 *Paroxysmal hemicrania*.
B. Not attributed to another disorder.

Probable SUNCT

The diagnostic criteria for probable SUNCT are given in Table 12.12.

Table 12.12   Diagnostic criteria for probable SUNCT

A. Attacks fulfilling all but one of criteria A–D for 3.3 *SUNCT*.
B. Not attributed to another disorder.

12.6 Differential diagnosis of 'TAC' and short-lasting headaches

The differences in diagnosis and treatment between 'TAC' and short-lasting headaches are listed in Table 12.13.

Table 12.13   Differences in diagnosis and treatment between 'TAC' and short-lasting headaches

	Cluster	EPH	CPH	SUNCT
Gender M : F	8 : 1	1 : 1	1 : 2	2–6 : 1
Pain description	Stabbing	Throbbing	Throbbing	Stabbing
Pain severity	Excruciating	Severe	Severe	Moderate
Attacks frequency	1 qod to 8 per day	2–30 per day	1–40 per day	30 per hour
Attacks duration	15–180 min	2–30 min	2–30 min	5–240 s
Treatment	Oxygen, triptan, verapamil, lithium	Indomethacin	Indomethacin	Lamotrigin, gabapentin, topiramate, lidocaine, corticosteroids

12.7 Other primary headaches

Other primary headaches include those shown in Table 12.14.

Table 12.14   Other primary headaches

4.1	Primary stabbing headache
4.2	Primary cough headache
4.3	Primary exertional headache
4.4	Primary headache associated with sexual activity
	4.4.1 Preorgasmic headache
	4.4.2 Orgasmic headache
4.5	Hypnic headache
4.6	Primary thunderclap headache
4.7	Hemicrania continua
4.8	New daily-persistent headache (NDPH)

General comment

Primary or secondary headache or both?

When a new headache occurs for the first time in close temporal relation to another disorder that is a known cause of headache, this headache is coded according to the causative disorder as a secondary headache. This is also true if the headache has the characteristics of migraine or other primary headache. When a pre-existing primary headache is made worse in close temporal relation to another disorder that is a known cause of headache, there are two possibilities and judgment is required. The patient can either be given only the diagnosis of the pre-existing primary headache or be given both this diagnosis and a secondary headache diagnosis according to the other disorder. Factors that support adding the latter diagnosis are a very close temporal relation to the disorder, a marked worsening of the pre-existing headache, very good evidence that the disorder can cause or aggravate the primary headache and, finally, improvement or resolution of the primary headache after relief from the disorder.

Introduction

These headaches are clinically heterogeneous. The pathogenesis of these types of headache is still poorly understood, and their treatment is suggested on the basis of anecdotal reports or uncontrolled trials. The onset of some of these headaches, 4.6 *Primary thunderclap headache* especially, can be acute, and affected patients are usually assessed in emergency departments. Appropriate and full investigation (neuroimaging in particular) is mandatory in these cases.

Primary stabbing headache

Details concerning primary stabbing headache are given in Table 12.15.

Table 12.15   Details concerning primary stabbing headache

Previously used terms
Ice-pick pains, jabs and jolts, ophthalmodynia periodica.

Description
Transient and localized stabs of pain in the head that occur spontaneously in the absence of organic disease of underlying structures or of the cranial nerves.

Diagnostic criteria
A. Head pain occurring as a single stab or a series of stabs and fulfilling criteria B–D.
B. Exclusively or predominantly felt in the distribution of the first division of the trigeminal nerve (orbit, temple and parietal area).
C. Stabs last for up to a few seconds and recur with irregular frequency ranging from one to many per day.
D. No accompanying symptoms.
E. Not attributed to another disorder.[1]

Note
1. History and physical and neurological examinations do not suggest any of the disorders listed in groups 5–12, or history and/or physical and/or neurological examinations do suggest such disorder but it is ruled out by appropriate investigations, or such disorder is present but pain does not occur for the first time in close temporal relation to the disorder.

Comments
In a single published descriptive study, 80% of stabs lasted 3 s or less. In rare cases, stabs occur repetitively over days, and there has been one description of status lasting 1 week.

Stabs may move from one area to another in either the same or the opposite hemicranium. When they are strictly localized to one area, structural changes at this site and in the distribution of the affected cranial nerve must be excluded. Stabbing pains are more commonly experienced by people subject to migraine (about 40%) or cluster headache (about 30%), in which cases they are felt in the site habitually affected by these headaches. A positive response to indomethacin has been reported in some uncontrolled studies, whilst others have observed partial or no responses.

Primary cough headache

Details concerning primary cough headache are given in Table 12.16.

Table 12.16 Details concerning primary cough headache

Previously used terms
Benign cough headache, Valsalva-maneuver headache.

Description
Headache precipitated by coughing or straining in the absence of any intracranial
  disorder.

Diagnostic criteria
A. Headache fulfilling criteria B and C
B. Sudden onset, lasting from one second to 30 min.
C. Brought on by and occurring only in association with coughing, straining and/or
    Valsalva maneuver.
D. Not attributed to another disorder.[1]

Note
1. Cough headache is symptomatic in about 40% of cases and the large majority of these
    present Arnold–Chiari malformation type I. Other reported causes of symptomatic
    cough headache include carotid or vertebrobasilar diseases and cerebral aneurysms.
    Diagnostic neuroimaging plays an important role in differentiating secondary cough
    headache from 4.2 Primary cough headache.

Comment
Primary cough headache is usually bilateral and predominantly affects patients older than
40 years of age. Whilst indomethacin is usually effective in the treatment of primary cough
headache, a positive response to this medication has also been reported in some symptomatic
cases.

Primary exertional headache

Details concerning primary exertional headache are given in Table 12.17.

Table 12.17 Details concerning primary exertional headache

Previously used terms
Benign exertional headache.

Coded elsewhere
Exercise-induced migraine is coded under 1. Migraine according to its subtype.

Description
Headache precipitated by any form of exercise. Subforms such as "weight-lifters' headache"
are recognized.

Table 12.17 *(continued)*

Diagnostic criteria
A. Pulsating headache fulfilling criteria B and C.
B. Lasting from 5 min to 48 h.
C. Brought on by and occurring only during or after physical exertion.
D. Not attributed to another disorder.[1]

Note
1. On first occurrence of this headache type it is mandatory to exclude subarachnoid hemorrhage and arterial dissection.

Comments
Primary exertional headache occurs particularly in hot weather or at high altitude. There are reports of prevention in some patients by the ingestion of ergotamine tartrate. Indomethacin has been found effective in the majority of the cases.

Headache described in weight-lifters has been considered a subform of 4.3 *Primary exertional headache*; because of its sudden onset and presumed mechanism it may have more similarities to 4.2 *Primary cough headache.*

Primary headache associated with sexual activity

Previously used terms   Benign sex headache, coital cephalalgia, benign vascular sexual headache, sexual headache.

Description   Headache precipitated by sexual activity, usually starting as a dull bilateral ache as sexual excitement increases and suddenly becoming intense at orgasm, in the absence of any intracranial disorder.

Preorgasmic headache

The diagnostic criteria for preorgasmic headache are listed in Table 12.18.

Table 12.18   Diagnostic criteria for orgasmic headache

A. Dull ache in the head and neck associated with awareness of neck and/or jaw muscle contraction and meeting criterion B.
B. Occurs during sexual activity and increases with sexual excitement.
C. Not attributed to another disorder.

Orgasmic headache

Details concerning orgasmic headache are given in Table 12.19.

Table 12.19   Details concerning orgasmic headache

Coded elsewhere
Postural headache resembling that of low cerebrospinal fluid (CSF) pressure has been reported to develop after coitus. Such headache should be coded as 7.2.3 *Headache attributed to spontaneous (or idiopathic) low CSF pressure* because it is due to CSF leakage.

Diagnostic criteria
A.   Sudden severe ('explosive') headache meeting criterion B.
B.   Occurs at orgasm.
C.   Not attributed to another disorder.[1]

Note
1.   On first onset of orgasmic headache it is mandatory to exclude conditions such as subarachnoid hemorrhage and arterial dissection.

Comments
An association between 4.4 *Primary headache associated with sexual activity*, 4.3 *Primary exertional headache* and migraine is reported in approximately 50% of cases.

Two subtypes (dull type and explosive type headache) were included in the first edition of The International Classification of Headache Disorders. No specific investigation has been undertaken since then to clarify whether they are separate entities. In most published reports of headache with sexual activity, only explosive ('vascular type') headache has been reported. The dull type may be a subtype of tension-type headache, but no evidence supports this hypothesis.

No firm data are available on the duration of primary headache associated with sexual activity, but it is usually considered to last from 1 min to 3 h.

Hypnic headache

Details concerning hypnic headache are given in Table 12.20.

Table 12.20   Details concerning hypnic headache

Previously used terms
Hypnic headache syndrome, 'alarm clock' headache.

Description
Attacks of dull headache that always awaken the patient from asleep.

Diagnostic criteria
A.   Dull headache fulfilling criteria B–D.
B.   Develops only during sleep and awakens patient.
C.   At least two of the following characteristics:
     1.   occurs >15 times per month

Table 12.20 *(continued)*

2. lasts $\geq$15 min after waking
3. first occurs after age of 50 years.
D. No autonomic symptoms and no more than one of nausea, photophobia or phonophobia.
E. Not attributed to another disorder.[1]

Note
1. Intracranial disorders must be excluded. Distinction from one of the TACs is necessary for effective management.

Comments
The pain of hypnic headache is usually mild to moderate, but severe pain is reported by approximately 20% of patients. Pain is bilateral in about two-thirds of cases. The attack usually lasts from 15 to 180 min, but longer durations have been described.

Caffeine and lithium have been effective treatments in several reported cases.

Primary thunderclap headache

Details concerning primary thunderclap headache are given in Table 12.21.

Table 12.21   Details concerning primary thunderclap headache

Previously used terms
Benign thunderclap headache.

Coded elsewhere
4.2 *Primary cough headache*, 4.3 *Primary exertional headache* and 4.4 *Primary headache associated with sexual activity* can all present as thunderclap headache but should be coded as those headache types, not as 4.6 *Primary thunderclap headache*.

Description
High-intensity headache of abrupt onset mimicking that of ruptured cerebral aneurysm.

Diagnostic criteria:
A. Severe head pain fulfilling criteria B and C.
B. Both of the following characteristics:
1. sudden onset, reaching maximum intensity in <1 min
2. lasting from 1 h to 10 days.
C. Does not recur regularly over subsequent weeks or months.[1]
D. Not attributed to another disorder.[2]

Notes
1. Headache may recur within the first week after onset.
2. Normal CSF and normal brain imaging are required.

Table 12.21 *(continued)*

Comment
Evidence that thunderclap headache exists as a primary condition is poor; the search for an underlying cause should be expedient and exhaustive. Thunderclap headache is frequently associated with serious vascular intracranial disorders, particularly subarachnoid hemorrhage; it is mandatory to exclude this and a range of other such conditions, including intracerebral hemorrhage, cerebral venous thrombosis, unruptured vascular malformation (mostly aneurysm), arterial dissection (intra- and extra-cranial), CNS angiitis, reversible benign CNS angiopathy and pituitary apoplexy. Other organic causes of thunderclap headache are colloid cyst of the third ventricle, CSF hypotension and acute sinusitis (particularly with barotrauma). 4.6 *Primary thunderclap headache* should be the diagnosis only when all organic causes have been excluded.

Hemicrania continua

Details concerning hemicrania continua are given in Table 12.22.

Table 12.22   Details concerning hemicrania continua

Description
Persistent strictly unilateral headache responsive to indomethacin.

Diagnostic criteria
A.   Headache for >3 months fulfilling criteria B–D.
B.   All of the following characteristics:
    1.   unilateral pain without side-shift
    2.   daily and continuous, without pain-free periods
    3.   moderate intensity, but with exacerbations of severe pain.
C.   At least one of the following autonomic features occurs during exacerbations and ipsilateral to the side of pain:
    1.   conjunctival injection and/or lacrimation
    2.   nasal congestion and/or rhinorrhea
    3.   ptosis and/or miosis.
D.   Complete response to therapeutic doses of indomethacin. Not attributed to another disorder.[1]

Note
1.   History and physical and neurological examinations do not suggest any of the disorders listed in groups 5–12, or history and/or physical and/or neurological examinations do suggest such disorder but it is ruled out by appropriate investigations, or such disorder is present but headache does not occur for the first time in close temporal relation to the disorder.

Comment
Hemicrania continua is usually unremitting, but rare cases of remission are reported. Whether this headache type can be subdivided according to length of history and persistence is yet to be determined.

References

1. Bahra, A., May, A. and Goadsby, P.J. (1999) Diagnostic patterns in cluster headache, in *Cluster Headache and Related Conditions* (eds J. Olesen and P.J. Goadsby), Oxford University Press, Oxford, pp. 61–65.

2. Goadsby, P.J. (2002) Pathophysiology of cluster headache: a trigeminal autonomic cephalgia. *Lancet Neurology*, **1** (4), 251–257.

3. Manzoni, G.C. (1998) Gender ratio of cluster headache over the years: a possible role of changes in lifestyle. *Cephalalgia: An International Journal of Headache*, **18**, 138–142.

4. May, A., Bahra, A., Buchel, C. *et al.* (1998) Hypothalamic activation in cluster headache attacks. *Lancet*, **351**, 275–278.

5. Torelli, P., Cologno, D., Cademartiri, C. and Manzoni, G.C. (2001) Application of the International Headache Society classification criteria in 652 cluster headache patients. *Cephalalgia: An International Journal of Headache*, **21**, 145–150.

6. Alberca, R. and Ochoa, J.J. (1994) Cluster tic syndrome. *Neurology*, **44**, 996–999.

7. Mulleners, W.M. and Verhagen, W.I.M. (1996) Cluster-tic syndrome. *Neurology*, **47**, 302.

8. Kudrow, L. (1980) *Cluster Headache: Mechanisms and Management*, Oxford University Press, Oxford.

9. Antonaci, F. and Sjaastad, O. (1989) Chronic paroxysmal hemicrania (CPH): a review of the clinical manifestations. *Headache*, **29**, 648–656.

10. Broeske, D., Lenn, N.J. and Cantos, E. (1993) Chronic paroxysmal hemicrania in a young child: possible relation to ipsilateral occipital infarction. *Journal of Child Neurology*, **8**, 235–236.

11. Headache Classification Subcommittee of the International Headache Society (2004) The International Classification of Headache Disorders: 2nd edition. *Cephalalgia*, **24** (Suppl 1), 1–160.

12. Antonaci, F., Pareja, J.A., Caminero, A.B. and Sjaastad, O. (1998) Chronic paroxysmal hemicrania and hemicrania continua. Parenteral indomethacin: the 'Indotest'. *Headache*, **38**, 122–128.

13. Kudrow, D.B. and Kudrow, L. (1989) Successful aspirin prophylaxis in a child with chronic paroxysmal hemicrania. *Headache*, **29**, 280–281.

14. Benoliel, R. and Sharav, Y. (1998) Trigeminal neuralgia with lacrimation or SUNCT syndrome? *Cephalalgia: An International Journal of Headache*, **18**, 85–90.

15. Bussone, G., Leone, M., Volta, G.D. *et al.* (1991) Short-lasting unilateral neuralgiform headache attacks with tearing and conjunctival injection: the first symptomatic case. *Cephalalgia: An International Journal of Headache*, **11**, 123–127.

16. Goadsby, P.J. and Lipton, R.B. (1997) A review of paroxysmal hemicranias, SUNCT syndrome and other short-lasting headaches with autonomic features, including new cases. *Brain: A Journal of Neurology*, **120**, 193–209.

17. Pareja, J.A. and Sjaastad, O. (1997) SUNCT syndrome. A clinical review. *Headache*, **37**, 195–202.

18. De Benedittis, G. (1996) SUNCT syndrome associated with cavernous angioma of the brain stem. *Cephalalgia: An International Journal of Headache,* **16**, 503–506.

19. Ferrari, M.D., Haan, J. and van Seters, A.P. (1988) Bromocriptine-induced trigeminal neuralgia attacks in a patient with pituitary tumor. *Neurology,* **38**, 1482–1484.

20. Massiou, H., Launay, J.M., Levy, C. *et al.* (2002) SUNCT syndrome in two patients with prolactinomas and bromocriptine-induced attacks. *Neurology,* **58**, 1698–1699.

21. Morales, F., Mostacero, E., Marta, J. and Sanchez, S. (1994) Vascular malformation of the cerebellopontine angle associated with SUNCT syndrome. *Cephalalgia: An International Journal of Headache,* **14**, 301–302.

13

Biobehavioral management of childhood headaches

Scott W. Powers

Incorporating a focus on health-promoting behaviors, adherence to recommended interventions and employment of nonpharmacological treatments into a comprehensive headache management plan is a key aspect of care for children with headaches. This chapter will discuss the application of lifestyle habits, pharmacological adherence and evidence-based nonpharmacological treatments to clinical practice.

13.1 Lifestyle habits

Changing and maintaining healthy lifestyle habits is central to pediatric headache care. Such lifestyle habits include regular sleep patterns, regular mealtimes, increased intake of green vegetables, regular exercise and increased intake of noncaffeinated liquids each day. Every child should receive these guidelines and, over the course of treatment, be assisted in making these changes and maintaining them as lifelong habits.

Specific recommendations are as follows:

- *Regular sleep.* There should be 8 to 10 h of sleep each night. Scheduling a similar bedtime and wake-up time each day is recommended. In order for this lifestyle habit to be maintained, some flexibility as to weekend sleep and wake times is incorporated into the recommendations. One common area of discussion pertains to wake-up time on Sunday mornings, with the goal that

Pediatric Headaches in Clinical Practice   Andrew D. Hershey, Paul Winner, Marielle A. Kabbouche and Scott W. Powers
© 2009 John Wiley & Sons, Ltd.

the child or adolescent is up at a time that makes going to sleep at the regular bedtime on Sunday night easy for them.

- *Regular mealtimes and increased intake of green vegetables.* Children and adolescents are encouraged to eat three meals at regular time intervals during the day and often to include one snack period after school. A variety of green vegetables and fruits are discussed with the children, and they are encouraged to increase their intake of those foods they already enjoy and to consider trying some foods they might not have sampled before. Food avoidance is not usually recommended.

- *Regular exercise.* Children and adolescents are asked to be generally active and to exercise at least three times a week for 30 min to the point of perspiring and exertion. Activities and exercises that the children find enjoyable and feasible during different seasons of the year and in their home and school environments should be discussed as part of the treatment planning process. Having fun with exercise is emphasized.

- *Adequate hydration.* Increased liquid intake of noncaffeinated beverages is a strong recommendation of a biobehavioral care program. Children and adolescents are encouraged to drink at least 2 L of liquids per day and to strive to intake 3 L of liquids per day during the summer and times of heavy exertion, such as sports activities. These liquids can include water, juice, milk and sports drinks. In a school note that should be given to children about their headache care, it is written that they can carry a water or sports drink bottle with them throughout the day to meet these increased liquid intake lifestyle goals.

During the course of treatment, children and their families and schools need help to make these changes. Also, via continuity of care, they need assistance with maintaining these behaviors as lifelong headache prevention and treatment strategies.

13.2 Pharmacologic adherence

Taking the right medication in the right dose at the right time is a critical headache care behavior. The child's role in recognizing the initial onset of a headache and telling a parent, teacher or other adult should be emphasized. This 'catch pain early' strategy is critical to the success of abortive pharmacologic treatment. In addition, the child's ability to name the abortive medication and the appropriate dose are key to their taking an active role in treating their headaches in various settings (e.g. home, school, during sports, at a friend's house). Children and adolescents also should be encouraged to drink 20 to 32 ounces of sports drink along with their medication at the onset of the headache. The child and their family need to be given a school letter indicating the exact name and dosage of their abortive medication treatment and stating that the prescription includes the intake of sports drink with the medication.

Similarly, taking prophylactic medication (if prescribed) as recommended is a critical headache care behavior. The preventive role of prophylactic medications should be emphasized with children and adolescents. This is done so that they can appreciate the difference between an abortive medication strategy and a preventive medication strategy. Developmentally and behaviorally, this concept is notable for children and adolescents. Specifically, abortive medication is taken at the moment of the onset of pain, whereas preventive medication is taken every day regardless of whether the child feels ill or not. This reasoning needs to be provided to children and reviewed to ensure developmentally appropriate and practical understanding.

Maintaining regular daily adherence to preventive medication is viewed as another central component of care for pediatric headache. Clarifying with children and adolescents the different roles of preventive and abortive medications and rehearsing with them the reasons for taking two different types of medication for their headaches is very beneficial to the long-term effectiveness of a headache treatment program. Finally, with regard to prophylactic medication, children and adolescents should be informed early in their treatment that, by implementing positive lifestyle habits and active abortive treatment approaches, it is likely they will not need to maintain long-term prescriptions of preventive medications. In our experience, we find that preventive medications, when prescribed, generally are not needed for more than a 6- to 12-month period for children diagnosed with headaches.

13.3 Nonpharmacological interventions

Pediatric headache care should include training children to use active coping skills. These coping skills include not only the aforementioned positive lifestyle habits and adherence to preventive and abortive medication regimens, but also evidence-based interventions, such as biofeedback-assisted relaxation training

(BART) [1]. Relaxation training usually involves one or more of the following techniques: progressive muscle relaxation, diaphragmatic or deep breathing, and guided imagery.

Progressive muscle relaxation training involves alternate tensing and relaxing of various muscle groups throughout the body. Its goal is to teach the child the contrast between tension and relaxation via systematic physical manipulation. Diaphragmatic or deep breathing involves systematic inhalation and exhalation. Again, the child learns the relationship between tension and relaxation by attention to breathing, which produces somatic changes in a systematic fashion. Guided imagery relies on a cognitive means of producing a state of relaxation. In this procedure, the child visualizes a pleasant scene or favored activity, such as playing in the woods or taking a ride on a favorite amusement park attraction, to achieve a state of relaxation. Even children who might not think that they like 'make-believe' can often readily engage in visualization, especially if their own ideas are involved in the development of the imagery script.

Relaxation training is used most often with children 7 years of age or older. However, with developmentally appropriate adjustments to the training procedures, relaxation training procedures, especially those emphasizing imagery, have been used successfully with preschool-age children and intellectually challenged children. In practice, because of the cognitive, attentional, social and emotional demands of the treatment, the use of standard relaxation training protocols is best suited for older children. Children need to be able to understand the rationale of using relaxation to combat feeling such severe pain. They also must be able to concentrate on their bodily sensations for an extended time and have the social and emotional maturity to learn both how to manage stress and how to sustain the practice necessary to acquire and maintain the relaxation.

Biofeedback is most often used as an adjunct to relaxation training to address headaches. Instrumentation is used to monitor the physiological effects of relaxation and/or to facilitate the learning of relaxation skills by providing visual and/or audio feedback about actual changes in otherwise invisible bodily processes. When described in this manner, it is evident that biofeedback itself is not a treatment modality. Rather, biofeedback instrumentation is used to enhance self-control and relaxation training. Therefore, in a biobehavioral approach to care, this technique can be referred to as BART.

In typical biofeedback for children and adolescents with headaches, two parameters considered correlates of physiologic arousal are the most commonly assessed. The first is electromyographic activity, electrical discharge in the muscle fibers, a correlate of skeletal muscle tension. The second parameter is peripheral skin temperature monitoring. Skin temperature is a correlate of vasomotor mechanisms. Feedback is usually given via a visual display on a computer screen. A line graph is a typical display, and displays for children can also be gamelike, using graphics and audio feedback. Biofeedback instrumentation is used in the relaxation treatment process to accomplish four goals: to make the child aware of physical responses; to teach children to control physiological responses; to enhance children's sense of self-control and self-efficacy (i.e. belief that they can do what they set out to do); and to transfer or generalize these skills to use in everyday life. Given that improvement in headache symptoms sometimes correlates better to enhancement of self-control and self-efficacy than to actual changes in physiology, these psychological variables may play an especially potent role.

When working with a provider of evidence-based, nonpharmacological interventions such as BART, children are introduced to the biofeedback equipment and given the rationale for its use. They are then asked to relax on their own as they normally would while their body's response is monitored. Then the children are taught deep-breathing skills and their physiologic responses are subsequently measured. Next, the child is taught progressive muscle relaxation. Electromyographic activity and peripheral temperature are monitored afterward. Third, the child is instructed in guided imagery using an individualized approach. Finally, a relaxation CD is made combining breathing, muscle relaxation and imagery exercises.

Children and adolescents who receive this treatment often exhibit a decrease in muscle tension and an increase in peripheral body temperature after this initial BART session. Such body changes are indications of a relaxation response. Specifically, the increase in peripheral body temperature has been associated with the prevention of headaches [2]. Children are able to show this response not only at initial training, but also 6 months later when they returned for a follow-up visit [3]. BART can also be utilized within an inpatient pediatric medical/surgical context by using portable biofeedback equipment which is easy to transport and operate. In our experience in an inpatient setting, where children typically do not have much control over their environment, schedule or interactions with people, biofeedback is often particularly welcomed. Children have expressed not only improvement in their physical symptoms, but also a return of a sense of control.

Children who receive BART are encouraged to practice with their relaxation CD three to five nights per week prior to bedtime for the first 2 weeks. Thereafter, they are encouraged to practice either with the CD or on their own three nights per week and at the onset of a headache. The relaxation CD is usually between 5 and 10 min in length. Children and adolescents often find these skills fun and useful. After a couple weeks of practice with the CD, most children find they can do this on their own and change their imagery as needed to keep the process from becoming monotonous. Children and adolescents also are encouraged to use relaxation skills any time they are experiencing stressors or challenges in their day-to-day lives.

13.4 Summary

In conclusion, biobehavioral treatment is a central feature of the care provided to children and adolescents with headache. Children and adolescents with headaches can be asked to behave in ways that optimize their control over their headaches. In addition, coping skills training that includes biofeedback-assisted relaxation skills is an efficacious and enjoyable adjunctive treatment for children and adolescents who experience headache disorders. These biobehavioral treatment approaches should be included in the interdisciplinary and comprehensive care of children seen for headaches [4]. Treatment programs for childhood headache could profit from incorporating this biobehavioral approach to care [5].

References

1. Eccleston, C., Yorke, L., Morley, S. *et al.* (2003) Psychological therapies for the management of chronic and recurrent pain in children and adolescents. *Cochrane Database of Systematic Reviews*, 1(Art. No.: CD003968), DOI: 10.1002/14651858.CD003968.

2. Hermann, C., Kim, M. and Blanchard, E.B. (1995) Behavioral and prophylactic pharmacological intervention studies of pediatric migraine: an exploratory meta-analysis. *Pain*, **60**, 239–255.

3. Powers, S.W., Mitchell, M.J., Byars, K.C. *et al.* (2001) A pilot study of one-session biofeedback training in pediatric headache. *Neurology*, **56**, 133.

4. Kabbouche, M., Powers, S.W., Vockell, A. *et al.* (2005) Outcome of a multidisciplinary approach to pediatric headache at 1, 2, and 5 years. *Headache*, **45**, 1298–1303.

5. Powers, S.W., Kruglak-Gilman, D. Hershey, A.D. and Headache Center Team at Cincinnati Children's Hospital (2006) Clinical Pearl/Brief Report: Suggestions for a biopsychosocial approach to treating children and adolescents who present with headache. *Headache*, **46**(Suppl. 3), S149–S150.

14

Sinus headache and nasal disease

Andrew D. Hershey

As noted previously in this text, headaches can be divided into primary headaches and secondary headaches. One of the most frequently diagnosed secondary headaches is sinus headaches or headaches attributed to rhinosinusitis (International Classification of Headache Disorders (ICHD)-II, 11.5) [1]. Patients frequently report sinus symptoms with their headaches, including rhinorrhea or nasal stuffiness, and often locate the pain in their 'sinuses'. Subsequently, either through self-diagnosis or practitioner diagnosis, they come to the conclusion that their headaches are caused by sinus disease. This is further complicated by a lack of a definitive diagnosis for sinusitis, although several different diagnoses have been developed. A detailed review of sinusitis and its etiologies can be found elsewhere [2]. This chapter will focus on the headache component and the symptomology.

14.1 Identification of sinus headache

The American Academy of Otolaryngology – Head and Neck Surgery (AAO-HNS) has developed working definitions for sinusitis, including acute, subacute and chronic [3]. The AAO-HNS working diagnosis of rhinosinusitis requires nasal endoscopy or computed tomography (CT) imaging of the paranasal sinuses for a definite diagnosis. Recognizing this limitation, a clinical diagnosis was also suggested. This clinical diagnosis included both major factors

Pediatric Headaches in Clinical Practice   Andrew D. Hershey, Paul Winner, Marielle A. Kabbouche and Scott W. Powers
© 2009 John Wiley & Sons, Ltd.

Table 14.1   AAO-HNS factors associated with rhinosinusitis [3]

Major factors
Purulence in nasal cavity
Facial pain, pressure, congestion or fullness
Nasal obstruction, blockage, discharge or purulence
Fever (acute)
Hyposmia or anosmia

Minor factors
Headache
Fever (non acute)
Halitosis
Fatigue
Dental Pain
Cough
Ear pain, pressure or fullness

---

and minor factors (Table 14.1). The presence of headache as a minor factor is where the confusion lies in separating a headache secondary to rhinosinusitis from a primary headache such as migraine or tension-type headache. This can be additionally complicated by AAO-HNS dividing the duration of the sinus symptoms, with acute being less than 4 weeks, subacute being 4–12 weeks and chronic being greater than 12 weeks.

As discussed throughout this text, ICHD-II serves as a reference for the diagnosis of headache disorders [1]. For sinus and related disorders this falls under the category of headache or facial pain contributed to disorders of the cranium, neck, eyes, ears, nose, sinuses, teeth, mouth or other facial or cranial structures with specifically headache attributed to rhinosinusitis falling under category 11.5 (Table 14.2). The hallmark of this diagnostic criterion is a frontal headache with laboratory imaging or clinical evidence consistent with acute or chronic rhinosinusitis. The pain is typically located over the involved sinus and its radiations. A timing component is also required to allow for the direct cause and effect of the sinus symptoms and headaches with a simultaneous onset, as well as resolution of headache with sinus symptoms and subsequent treatment. Of particular note, only acute sinusitis is noted to be attributed to headaches, with chronic sinusitis not felt to have a direct correlation unless there is an acute exacerbation.

ICHD-II further stresses that what is typically classified as a 'sinus headache' is oftentimes a misdiagnosis of migraine or tension-type headaches and clarifies

Table 14.2 ICHD-II criteria for headache attributed to rhinosinusitis. (ICHS II criteria from *Cephalalgia* 2004: 24 (Suppl 1): 1–160)

A.	Frontal headache accompanied by pain in one or more regions of the face, ears or teeth and fulfilling criteria C and D.
B.	Clinical, nasal endoscopic, CT and/or magnetic resonance imaging and/or laboratory evidence of acute or acute-on-chronic rhinosinusitis.
C.	Headache and facial pain develop simultaneously with onset of acute exacerbation of rhinosinusitis.
D.	Headache and/or facial pain resolve within 7 days after remission of successful treatment of acute or acute-on-chronic rhinosinusitis.

Notes
1. Clinical evidence may include purulence in the nasal cavity, nasal obstruction, hyposmia/anosmia and/or fever.
2. Chronic sinusitis is not validated as a cause of headache or facial pain unless relapsing into an acute stage.

appropriate diagnosis; the headache should be diagnosed as headache directly attributed to rhinosinusitis disease.

14.2 Epidemiology

The epidemiology of headache attributed to rhinosinusitis is complex due to this confusion with primary headache disorders. Several studies have been conducted to attempt to address this issue and clarify the diagnosis of migraine where sinus symptoms are present. One of the largest studies in the epidemiology of headache in the United States was the American Migraine Study II [4]. In this study, it was estimated that nearly 42% of patients with migraine that met ICHD-I [5] had been diagnosed previously by a physician with sinus headaches. This observation of the potential misdiagnosis of migraine as sinus headache led the investigators to examine the diagnosis of sinus headache in population and practitioner-assigned studies.

A small study conducted in 2002 in 47 patients who had a self-diagnosis of sinus headaches found that 90% of these patients had headaches at one time that met ICDH-I for migraine [6]. Furthermore, the most effective treatment for these patients was migraine-related therapies, and it was concluded that the rhinosinus symptoms reported by these patients were features of their migraine attacks.

Further expanding on this observation, 2991 patients in 452 primary care offices with a self-described or a physician-diagnosed sinus headache were assessed for their headache diagnosis using ICDH-I [7]. The age ranged studied was 18 to 65 years and the patients were required to have recurrent headaches with at least six headaches in the 6 months prior to the interview. Many of these patients reported sinus symptoms during their headaches, including sinus pressure in 84%, sinus pain in 82% and nasal congestion in 63%. In addition, many migraine features were also noted in this group of patients, with moderate to severe pain in nearly all of the patients (97%), a pulsatile quality of the pain in 89%, the presence of photophobia in 79% and phonophobia in 67%. Furthermore, 28% of the patients reported having an aura preceding their headaches and nausea occurred in 73% with vomiting in 24%. When these headache features were combined, 80% of the patients met ICDH-I for migraine with an additional 8% having migrainous headaches. An additional 8% had episodic tension-type headaches and only 4% were categorized as other type of headache.

A prospective study examining this potential misdiagnosis (the Sinus, Allergy, and Migraine Headache Study) investigated 100 consecutive patients responding to a newspaper advertisement for sinus headaches [8]. The research subjects volunteering for this study had a detailed history, and examination focused on using ICHD-I for headache diagnosis. After a detailed review, 63% of the subjects had migraine, 23% had migrainous headache/probable migraine and only 3% had a secondary headache attributed to rhinosinusitis, with 9% of the subjects not being able to be classified by ICDH-I. This study further examined the reasons why their was such a misdiagnosis by the patients or practitioners; the most common reason was location of the pain in 98%, with rhinorrhea in 73% and headaches induced by weather changes (83%), seasonal changes (73%) or allergens (62%) that led to the conclusion that the headache was an allergic sinus headache.

An alternative way to examine this issue is the presence of headache seen in a rhinology or ENT clinic for a referral of sinus headache [9]. An analysis of 100 consecutive patients that presented to a tertiary rhinology practice for rhino-sinusitis with no CT evidence of acute sinus disease were examined for the headache etiology [9]. This analysis included the use of the Sino-Nasal Outcome Test (SNOT-20). This is a 20-item questionnaire that assesses facial pain, headache and other symptomology. The patients were divided into three groups: Group I – specifically had headache or facial pain as their chief complaint of their symptoms (36 patients); Group II – headache was only one of the constellations of the symptoms (33 patients); and Group III – no headache (31 patients). If the patients did have severe headaches (Group I), then the patient was referred for subsequent neurological evaluation. Of the Group I patients, 21 of the 36 patients were diagnosed on neurological examination as having migraine with five having nonspecific headache, four having 'rebound headache', and two having tension-type headaches. In addition, the patients in Group I had the highest SNOT-20 scores and reflected a higher degree of pain, disability and impact on quality of life. With the lack of significant rhinosinusitis symptoms, their conclusion was that the most likely diagnosis is migraine and that, when patients present with complaint of sinus headache, a brief 20-point questionnaire would be able to differentiate those that need further referral.

14.3 Sinus headache diagnosis

As noted above, the AAO-HNS established criteria for the diagnosis of rhinosinusitis (Table 14.1) and ICDH-II established fine criteria for headache attributed to rhinosinusitis (Table 14.2). In order to differentiate headache attributed to rhinosinusitis from primary headaches, key features may assist in separating those headaches that are due to rhinosinusitis and those headaches that are due to migraine. Although many of the symptoms overlap, making it difficult in separating sinus headache from migraine, there may be some distinguishing features. For most patients with clearly identified headache attributed to rhinosinusitis, sinus-related pain appears to be a pressure-like pain that was dull, may be bilateral and is usually periorbital, although it can be unilateral. It is typically worse in the morning and improves as the day progresses, indicating a possibility of sinus frame age in the upright position. There may be signs of nasal obstruction or congestion that may last days at a time and which usually are not associated with the typical features of migraine, including nausea, vomiting, auras, photophobia or phonophobia. There is some suggestion that change in atmospheric pressure or sinus pressure can have worsening symptoms. One such test is the Mueller sign. In this procedure, the patient pinches their nose shut, blows their nose hard to pressurize their sinuses, and then coughs. A positive finding in this is a localized pain over the infected sinus upon the cough maneuver.

Migraine, on the other hand, has its own distinct diagnoses that differentiate from above. In a migraine patient there may be sinus pressure, sinus pain and nasal congestion; but, in addition, there are migraine-specific symptoms. The presence of these migraine-specific symptoms, including moderate to severe pain, pulsatile quality, photophobia, phonophobia and nausea and/or vomiting, make the diagnosis of migraine more likely. Differentiating the sinus headaches from migraine is the most essential component to make the proper treatment, and when this continues to be difficult to ascertain, then imaging studies or nasal endoscopy may be necessary.

14.4 Treatment

When acute rhinosinusitis or chronic rhinosinusitis is highly suspected, treatment of the sinus symptoms should be initiated. These need to be specific for treating the underlying etiology and can include allergy-specific medications, including nasal steroid sprays or systemic decongestants, as well as antibiotic therapy. Adequate trials of these medications are essential to assure that the sinus symptoms have been treated. Once this adequate trial has been attained, a re-examination for the continued presence of headaches and sinus symptoms is made. Oftentimes, the sinus symptoms will have resolved but the intermittent headaches will persist. In the presence of chronic daily headaches, this can be further confusing, as the headache has intermittent exacerbations but may have sinus qualities. In addition, if the allergy symptoms are a triggering factor for the migraines, then the patient may have a false impression of response to allergy treatment while continuing to have their episodic headaches but at a lower rate. Therefore, it is essential with treatment to have ongoing evaluations for the changing pattern and description of the headache characteristics. When there is no evidence of acute sinus or sinusitis symptoms, then treatment for migraine with migraine-specific medications should first be initiated.

14.5 Summary

In summary, for headache attributed to rhinosinusitis, the key components differentiating between sinus headaches and migraine are:

1. A recurrent pattern of headaches is suggestive of migraine, whereas an acute exacerbation or an acute new headache may be suggestive of headache secondary to rhinosinusitis.

2. Headaches that are self-limited and of brief duration (i.e. less than days) with clear nasal discharge may also represent a migraine-like phenomenon.

3. If rhinosinusitis symptoms are a predominant factor, then a careful evaluation by ENT may be necessary to identify particular pathology and possible treatment initiation.

4. In the presence of fever during a headache attack, rhinosinusitis should be considered. Of note, young children may have a low-grade fever during their migraine attacks.

5. An adequate course of treatment and detailed evaluations and follow-up are necessary to separate the two disorders for appropriate long-term outcome and benefit. With persistent headache and additional symptoms, further evaluation may be necessary.

14.6 Other nasal diseases and headache

For children and adolescents, the most typical presentation of headache associated with nasal and sinus-related disease is primary headache or headache attributed to rhinosinusitis as discussed above; contact-point headaches also can occur, causing facial pain but without sinus infection. The etiology of this disorder can be due to anatomical pathology in the nasal cavity that is traumatic, is acquired secondary to other disease states or is congenital. This can include sinus polyps, nasal septal spurs and abnormalities of the tribunates. The source of the pain is abnormal contact of the nasal mucosa triggering the pain. One such type of contact headache in which the there is an enlargement of the middle turbinate has been called concha bullosa [10].

The prevalence of these conditions has not been well characterized, but may be frequently observed in sinus CT examinations [11]. It is not known how often this abnormality contributes to headache or facial pain in children. When there is a clinical presentation of a periorbital or mid-canthal pain that may

Table 14.3 Mucosal contact point headache. (ICHD-II criteria reproduced with permission from Blackwell Publishing)

A. Intermittent pain localized to the periorbital and medial canthal or temporozygomatic regions and fulfilling criteria C and D.

B. Clinical, nasal endoscopic and/or CT imaging evidence of mucosal contact points without acute rhinosinusitis

C. Evidence that the pain can be attributed to mucosal contact based on at least one of the following:
   (i)   pain corresponds to gravitational variations in mucosal congestion as the patient moves between upright and recumbent postures;
   (ii) abolition of pain within 5 min after diagnostic topical application of local anesthesia to the middle turbinate using placebo or other controls.

D. Pain resolves within 7 days, and does not recur, after surgical removal of mucosal contact point.

spread to the temporal region with typically pain under the eyes and a lack of the associated symptoms typical of migraine, this diagnosis should be entertained and a sinus CT may be revealing. ICDH-II has specific criteria in the appendix as outlined in Table 14.3 for mucosal contact-point headaches (ICHD-II, A11.5.1). Contact-point headaches oftentimes need surgical treatment before resolution of headache symptoms.

References

1. Headache Classification Subcommittee of the International Headache Society (2004) The International Classification of Headache Disorders. *Cephalagia*, **24**(Suppl. 1), 1–160.
2. Piccirillo, J.F. (2004) Clinical practice. Acute bacterial sinusitis. *The New England Journal of Medicine*, **351**(9), 902–910.
3. Lanza, D.C. and Kennedy, D.W. (1997) Adult rhinosinusitis defined. *Otolaryngology and Head and Neck Surgery*, **117**(3), (Pt 2), S1–S7.
4. Lipton, R.B., Diamond, S., Reed, M. *et al.* (2001) Migraine diagnosis and treatment: results from the American Migraine Study II. *Headache*, **41**(7), 638–645.
5. Headache Classification Committee of the International Headache Society (1988) Classification and diagnostic criteria for headache disorders, cranial neuralgias and facial pain. *Cephalalgia: An International Journal of Headache*, **8** (Suppl 7), 1–96.
6. Lipton, R.B., Stewart, W.F. and Liberman, J.N. (2002) Self-awareness of migraine: interpreting the labels that headache sufferers apply to their headaches. *Neurology*, **58**(9), (Suppl. 6), S21–S26.
7. Schreiber, C.P., Hutchinson, S., Webster, C.J. *et al.* (2004) Prevalence of migraine in patients with a history of self-reported or physician-diagnosed 'sinus' headache. *Archives of Internal Medicine*, **164**(16), 1769–1772.
8. Eross, E.J., Dodick, D.W. and Eross, M.D. (2004) The Sinus, Allergy and Migraine Study (SAMS). *Headache*, **44**, 462.
9. Perry, B.F., Login, I.S. and Kountakis, S.E. (2004) Nonrhinologic headache in a tertiary rhinology practice. *Otolaryngology and Head and Neck Surgery*, **130**(4), 449–452.
10. Blaugrund, S.M. (1989) Nasal obstruction. The nasal septum and concha bullosa. *Otolaryngologic Clinics of North America*, **22**(2), 291–306.
11. Goldsmith, A., Zahtz, G., Stegnjajic, A. and Shikowitz, M. (1993) Middle turbinate headache syndrome. *American Journal of Rhinology*, **7**, 17–23.

15
Posttraumatic headaches

Paul Winner

Children who are involved in motor vehicle accidents, bicycle accidents and sports-related injuries, as well as head injuries secondary to child abuse, may develop a headache syndrome within 24 h to weeks following the incident, even after what would seem to be a trivial head injury. Most children who are hospitalized following a head injury have a Glasgow coma scale between 13 and 15 (Table 15.1). Patients who have Glasgow coma scales of <8 account for approximately 5% of hospital admissions.

Headaches in children that occur following a minor head injury often clear within 2 to 3 months. Headache and the constellation of symptoms that occur following trauma are sometimes referred to as posttraumatic or postconcussion syndrome. The associated symptoms may include vertigo, dizziness, difficulty concentrating, memory disorders, altered school performance, behavior disorders and sleep alteration [1–3]. Unfortunately, the pathophysiology of posttraumatic headache and postconcussion syndrome following a minor head injury is not as well understood as that which occurs following a severe head injury. The severity of the symptoms does not seem to depend on the severity of the head injury. Severe headaches, impaired memory and difficulty concentrating have been reported with both severe and relatively minor head injuries [4]. The headaches associated with the postconcussion syndrome can be similar to a migraine, a tension-type headache or both. Other rare, even cluster-type, headaches have been reported following a head injury [5]. Children without concussion symptoms and mild head injury with Glasgow coma scales of 13 to 15 may have symptoms ranging from no detectable structural abnormality to focal periangular brain lesions or dural hemorrhages.

Pediatric Headaches in Clinical Practice   Andrew D. Hershey, Paul Winner, Marielle A. Kabbouche and Scott W. Powers
© 2009 John Wiley & Sons, Ltd.

Table 15.1   Glasgow coma scale

Eye opening
   Spontaneous 4
   To sound 3
   To pain 2
   None 1
Verbal response
   Oriented 5
   Confused 4
   Inappropriate 3
   Incomprehensible 2
   None 1
Best motor response
   Obeys 6
   Localizes 5
   Withdraws 4
   Abnormal flexion 3
   Extends 2
   None 1

The clinical and neurobehavioral abnormalities following mild head injury have been fairly well established using a monkey model for a minor acceleration/deceleration nonimpact head injury in the sagittal plane wherein the animal sustained a brief loss of consciousness but no reported neurologic deficits [6]. Degenerating axons were noted in the pons and dorsal midbrain 7 days postinjury. Injuries in experimental animals and humans suggest that trauma causes a disorganization of the neurofilament cytoskeleton and axolemma and results in axonal disconnection [7]. A minor acceleration/deceleration injury that involves rotational forces may result in axonal shearing or tearing, especially in areas of the midbrain, superior cerebellar peduncles, corpus callosum and central white matter of the brain [8]. Acceleration/deceleration of the brain may also damage the labyrinth and mechanoreceptor in the neck and central vestibular connections, resulting in the symptoms of dizziness and vertigo that are often reported by patients with postconcussion syndrome. Blood vessels may be stretched or injured during the head injury; this impairs the vascular contractility in autoregulation that may result from direct vascular damage or may be a residual from tissue injury. Acceleration/deceleration forces may also result in stretch and strain of the cervical ligaments and muscles and the supporting bony structures of the neck [9].

Postconcussion syndrome symptoms seem to be more common after a mild to moderate head injury than after a severe head injury. It is important to note that direct impact is not necessary for the development of a postconcussion syndrome [10]. The unsynchronized rotational forces that may develop between the cerebral hemisphere in the cerebellum and the axons in the upper brain stem are more vulnerable to diffuse axonal injury; this may play a role in explaining the symptom complex that develops following head injury. The persistence of headache and associated symptoms may not correlate with the duration of unconsciousness, posttraumatic amnesia or skull fracture. A concussion produced by rotational forces to a semisolid brain within a skull can give rise to shearing and diffuse axonal injury [7]. This correlation with clinical symptomatology needs to be addressed further. Clearly, further work is necessary to understand the pathophysiology and clinical relationship of this information

15.1 Diagnostic issues

By gaining a greater understanding of the neurophysiology of head injuries, our understanding of the pathophysiology of head pain and its associated symptom complex will increase (Table 15.2). The guidelines established by the International Headache Society require headache onset to occur within 2 weeks of either the head injury or the time the patient regains consciousness in order to be considered a posttraumatic injury. This appears to be a reasonable guide, although patients may report headache onset as long as 1 month after the injury. This may be due to the fact that other injuries were sustained or other symptoms were more distressing.

Some patients report migraine-like headache symptoms following the injury; however, these headaches often do not respond well to standard migraine medications [11–13]. The neurologic sequelae of mild head injuries in children who report headache include hyperactivity, difficulty concentrating, memory

Table 15.2 Posttraumatic headache

Begins in days or weeks
Migraine headache-like quality
Cognitive difficulties
Symptoms may not equal injury
Subsides spontaneously in the majority of children

disorders, vertigo, dizziness, depression and altered personality causing altered school performance and behavior disorders [14, 15]. Both the patient and the family must be assured that the associated symptoms are common but will probably resolve over the next several weeks to months, although this may not be true for all children. The problem lies in determining which children will and will not fully recover.

Patients under the age of 12 years who have a sports-related injury rarely sustain a severe brain injury [16]. The potential for long-term sequelae following minor head injury in young athletes is unknown. There are concerns regarding second-impact syndrome. In this situation, a young athlete with a minor head injury recovers uneventfully; however, if the child sustains another minor head injury some time within the next week, then rapid cerebral edema could occur, resulting in death [17]. There may be issues related to the sequential minor injuries to the brain with resultant cerebral swelling and diminished intracranial compliance. Thus, the issue of when an athlete can return to play following a minor head injury is controversial, and new guidelines have been proposed [18]. Headaches in children may be caused by idiopathic intracranial hypertension (pseudotumor cerebri) with or without papilledema, minor head injury, carotid sheath injury and temporomandibular injury.

Table 15.3 The International Classification of Headache Disorders-II classification:[a] headache attributed to head and neck trauma

---

1. Acute posttraumatic headache
   1.1 Acute posttraumatic headache attributed to moderate or severe head injury
   1.2 Acute posttraumatic headache attributed to mild head injury
2. Chronic posttraumatic headache
   2.1 Chronic posttraumatic headache attributed to moderate or severe head injury
   2.2 Chronic posttraumatic headache attributed to mild head injury
3. Acute headache attributed to whiplash injury
4. Chronic headache attributed to whiplash injury
5. Headache attributed to traumatic intracranial hematoma
   5.1 Headache attributed to epidural hematoma
   5.2 Headache attributed to subdural hematoma
6. Headache attributed to other head and/or neck trauma
   6.1 Acute headache attributed to other head and/or neck trauma
   6.2 Chronic headache attributed to other head trauma
7. Postcraniotomy headache
   7.1 Acute postcraniotomy headache
   7.2 Chronic postcraniotomy headache

---

[a] Reproduced from Ref. [48].

Temporomandibular disorder may be a headache trigger [19]. Some children report sleep disturbances, including insomnia, daytime drowsiness, nonspecific staring episodes, periodic loss of consciousness, neurocognitive deficits and an inability to process information [20] (Table 15.3).

15.2 Considerations for returning to play after a concussion injury

The child is recommended to be removed from the activity; an individual may return to play in 1 week after a grade 1 (mild) concussion or one grade 2 (moderate) concussion. The individual may return to play in 2 weeks after multiple grade 2 concussions. However, after a grade 3 (severe) concussion, return to play should be delayed for 1 month or longer (consider termination for the remainder of the season), based on the judgment of the evaluating physician [21]. Note that the final recommendations should be rendered by the treating physician. For example, if a child had a grade 2 concussion, that would require a 1–2-week absence from sports. Most posttraumatic headaches resolve within 3 months.

There are different options in regard to when a patient should return to sporting activities. There are published guidelines in the sports medicine literature, but their success has not been confirmed. Certainly, departing from published guidelines on the basis of clinical judgment may be appropriate in individual cases [21].

The following are suggested guidelines for return to play after a grade 1 (mild) concussion. After the first concussion, the player may return to play if they have been asymptomatic for 1 week. After the second concussion, the player may return to play in 2 weeks if they have been asymptomatic at that time for 1 week. After the third concussion, the player's season shall be terminated; the player may return to play the next season if asymptomatic [21].

The following are suggested guidelines for return to play after a grade 2 (moderate) concussion. After the first concussion, the player may return to play after being asymptomatic for 1 week. After the second concussion, the player should stay off the field for a minimum of 1 month; they may then return to play if asymptomatic for at least 1 week and should consider terminating the season. After the third concussion, the player's season should be terminated, but the player may return to play the next season if they are symptomatic [21].

The following are suggested guidelines for return to play after a grade 3 (severe) concussion. After the first concussion, the player should stay off the field for a minimum of 1 month; they may then return to play after being asymptomatic for 1 week. After the second concussion, the player's season should be terminated; the player may return to play the next season if asymptomatic [21].

15.3 Evaluations

Most children who are hospitalized for a mild to moderate head injury receive some form of neuroimaging, either computed tomography (CT) or magnetic resonance imaging (MRI). The absence of abnormality on MRI or CT does not predict whether a patient will develop posttraumatic headaches or postconcussion syndrome. Patients who have a mild behavior abnormality and a Glasgow coma scale of <15 should have an MRI of the brain to rule out chronic subdural hematoma, hydrocephalus or a structural lesion unrelated to the trauma [22]. If a patient has associated cervical symptoms, then an MRI of the cervical region should be obtained. Initial studies suggest that single photon emission CT (SPECT) imaging may be helpful in predicting central nervous system (CNS) outcomes [23–25]. Early assessments indicate that SPECT scans may be somewhat more sensitive as long-term outcome predictors than CT or MRI scans [26].

Brain stem auditory-evoked potentials have been found to be abnormal in 10–20% of individuals with head-injury-associated postconcussion syndrome [22]. This relationship and its usefulness as a predictor for postconcussion sequelae need further assessment.

15.4 Neuropsychologic testing

Children with postconcussion syndrome may have abnormalities in information processing, auditory vigilance, reaction time, attention, visual and verbal memory, and analytic capacity [27]. Following mild head injury, there seems to be a hierarchy of functional recovery in those individuals who do recover, which is fortunately the vast majority of children.

Attention and concentration deficits usually resolve within 6 to 8 weeks. Visual memory, imagination, and analytic capacity also resolve, but not within 6 weeks. Verbal memory, abstraction, cognitive selectivity, and information processing speed may take more than 12 weeks to recover [27]. Migraine, tension-type, cluster, and chronic daily headache patterns have all been reported in patients with minor head injury [28, 29].

Patients who reported posttraumatic headaches commonly had a prior history of headache [30, 31]. Although many children have clinical improvement of their headache sequelae within several weeks to months, although some patients never have complete recovery with regard to headache and the associated symptoms of postconcussion syndrome. Patients have been reported to have continuing symptoms, which are independent of financial compensation, for 3 to 5 years after the injury [32–34]. The formal diagnosis of posttraumatic headaches and postconcussion syndrome requires that the constellation of symptoms is present and its onset is related to the head trauma.

Head injury accounts for the largest number of emergency department visits by children [35]. Subdural hemorrhage, cerebral vein thrombosis, cavernous sinus thrombosis, carotid artery dissection, epilepsy, cerebral hemorrhage, CNS neoplasm, and hydrocephalus must be ruled out [21].

15.5 Management

Children with head injury require rapid clinical assessment, as well as anticipation of the potential for intracranial complications. Patients with posttraumatic headaches are often misdiagnosed or undiagnosed, and parents of children may dismiss the complaints as being just a headache. The issue may be further complicated if other associated symptoms of postconcussion syndrome are present and undiagnosed. Thus, the most beneficial approach is to educate the parents and the child as to what potentially may occur. Simply discussing what posttraumatic headache and postconcussion syndrome are and what may occur in the next several weeks and months may be therapeutic.

The initial headache symptoms and soft-tissue injuries may be effectively treated with mild analgesics and nonsteroidal anti-inflammatory drugs (NSAIDs) over the initial several weeks. When cervical soft-tissue symptoms are present, a short course of physical therapy might be of benefit, depending on the patient's age and circumstances. If more prominent associated symptoms of anxiety, depression or cognitive difficulties are present, then more aggressive intervention may be necessary. Posttraumatic headache usually responds to the medications that are used for chronic daily headache and chronic tension-type headache, although no specific medication or treatment protocol has been found that will alter the underlying CNS disturbance.

Tricyclic antidepressants, such as amitriptyline (Elavil) or nortriptyline (Pamelor), are often the medications of choice. In children, the cardiac side effects are of concern. The beta-blockers may also prove helpful, although these drugs may potentiate fatigue or produce depression. Cyproheptadine, a drug that produces sedation, may be helpful, especially for patients with sleep disorders, since it can be given as a single nighttime dose. If patients are having frequent headaches, then it is important to talk about medication overuse or the possibility of developing rebound headaches. Analgesic use should be limited to no more than twice a week. NSAID use should be limited to two to three times a week, since these drugs have the potential to cause rebound headaches. The NSAIDs have potential gastrointestinal and renal side effects and need to be carefully monitored if they are to be used long term.

Children who have migraine-like posttraumatic headaches may benefit from triptans, with or without antiemetics. If must be noted that triptans and the majority of the medications used are not Food and Drug Administration approved for use in the age group. Some patients may respond to dihydroergotamine (DHE 45), especially if a refractory headache pattern persists. Nonpharmacologic therapies, such as biofeedback and stress management techniques, can be quite effective, even in children as young as 9 years of age [14]. It is important that teachers and other family members be aware of postconcussion syndrome and its potential sequelae, especially when children are having difficulty in school following a minor head injury. A psychologist may be helpful for teaching older children coping mechanisms for pain. If symptoms do not resolve by 6 months, then physiologic testing should be considered and medication regimens reassessed [36].

It was formerly believed that young children are less vulnerable to long-term sequelae of brain injury than older children. Recent research does not support the concept that younger brains recover better or more comprehensively after injury [37]. Differences based on focal lesions are not consistently seen, and younger brains do not appear to recover better than those of older children [38–40]. Present knowledge regarding the relationship between age and CNS injury outcome is quite complex and depends on a variety of factors involving the nature and timing of the injury and the environmental contacts [41]. It is believed that the developing brain is more vulnerable to cerebral injury than the fully developed brain [42]. Present evidence suggests that outcomes following minor head injuries are similar in adults and children [43, 44].

Owing to the fact that different definitions of head injury and different study designs have been used, it is difficult to ascertain the prognosis of posttraumatic headache in the studies available. At 1 month after mild head injury, as many as 90% of adult patients reported headache [45]; 2 to 3 months post-injury, as many as 78% reported headache [15]. At 1 year post-injury, 35–54% of patients reported headache symptoms [46]. At 2–4 years after injury, 20–24% of patients reported persistent headache symptoms.

Approximately one-third of adults are unable to return to work after a head injury [47]. The data in children are unclear.

15.6 Conclusions

Presently, there are no precise criteria for predicting the clinical outcome of children following head injury. The headache and associated symptoms usually gradually improve over a period of 3–6 months. Children who experience persistent symptoms that do not abate over the course of months to years are believed to have sustained a diffuse injury resulting from acceleration/deceleration forces. Children may benefit from a combination of pharmacologic and nonpharmacologic therapies for symptomatic relief.

References

1. Evans, R.W. (1992) The postconcussion syndrome and the sequelae of mild head injury. *Neurologic Clinics*, **10**, 815–847.
2. Rizzo, M. and Tranel, D. (1993) *Pediatric Trauma*, Mosby, Eichelberge, pp. 352–361.
3. Goldstein, B. and Powers, K.S. (1994) Head trauma in children. *Pediatrics in Review*, **15**, 213–219.
4. Rizzo, M. and Tranel, D. (1996) *Head Injury and Postconcussive Syndrome*, Churchill Livingston, New York, pp. 51–52.
5. Reik, L. (1987) Cluster headache after head injury. *Headache*, **27**, 509–510.
6. Jane, J.A., Steward, O. and Gennarelli, T. (1985) Axonal degeneration induced by experimental noninvasive minor head injury. *Journal of Neurosurgery*, **62**, 96–100.
7. Christman, C.W., Grady, M.S., Walker, S.A. *et al.* (1994) Ultrastructural studies of diffuse axonal injury in humans. *Journal of Neurotrauma*, **11**, 173–186.
8. Rizzo, M. and Tranel, D. (1996) *Head Injury and Postconcussive Syndrome*, Churchill Livingston, New York, p. 55.
9. Gordon, B. (1990) Postconcussional syndrome, in *Current Therapy in Neurologic Disease* (ed. R.T. Johnson), B.C. Decker, Philadelphia, pp. 208–213.
10. Gennarelli, T.A. (1993) Mechanisms of brain injury. *Journal of Emergency Medicine*, **1**, 511.
11. Evans, R.W. (1992) The postconcussion syndrome and the sequelae of mild head injury. *Neurologic Clinics*, **10**, 815–847.
12. Mandel, S. (1989) Minor head injury may not be "minor". *Postgraduate Medicine*, **85**, 213–215.
13. Brenner, C., Friendman, A.P., Merritt, H.H. *et al.* (1944) Post-traumatic headache. *Journal of Neurosurgery*, **1**, 317–391.
14. Winner, P. (1999) Post-traumatic headache, in *Current Management in Child Neurology* (ed. B.L. Maria), B.C. Decker, Hamilton, ON, pp. 57–58.

15. Rimel, R.W, Giordani, B., Barth J.T. *et al.* (1981) Disability caused by minor head injury. *Neurosurgery*, **9**(3), 221–228.

16. Bruce, D.A., Schut, L. and Sutton, L.N. (1982) Brain and cervical spine injuries occurring during organized sports activities in children and adolescents. *Clinics in Sports Medicine*, **1**, 495–514.

17. Saudners, R.L. and Harbaugh, R.E. (1984) The second impact in catastrophic contact-sports head trauma. *The Journal of the American Medical Association*, **252**, 538–539.

18. Rizzo, M. and Tranel, D. (1996) *Head Injury and Postconcussive Syndrome*, Churchill Livingston, New York, p. 449.

19. Silberstein, S. and Marcelis, J. (1990) Pseudotumor cerebri without papilledema. *Headache*, **30**, 304.

20. Gronwall, D. and Wrightston, P. (1974) Delayed recovery of intellectual function after minor head injury. *Lancet*, **2**, 605–609.

21. Cerhan, J., Shapiro, E. and Kriel, R. (1996) Neurologic and neuropsychological aspects of minor head injury in children, in *Head Injury and Postconcussive Syndrome* (eds M. Rizzo and D. Tranel), Churchill Livingstone, New York, pp. 448–449.

22. Silberstein, S., Lipton, R. and Goadsby, P. (1998) Post-traumatic headache, in *Headache in Clinical Practice* (eds S. Silberstein, R. Lipton and P. Goadsby), Oxford University Press, Corby, p. 139.

23. Abdel-Dayem, H.M., Sadek, S.A., Kouris, K. *et al.* (1987) Changes in cerebral perfusion after acute head injury: comparison of CT with Tc-99m HM-PAO SPECT. *Radiology*, **165**, 221–226.

24. Reid, R.H., Gulenchyn, K.Y., Ballinger, J.R. and Ventureyra, E.C. (1990) Cerebral perfusion imaging with technetium-99m HMPAO following cerebral trauma. Initial experience. *Clinical Nuclear Medicine*, **15**, 383–388.

25. Abdel-Dayem, H., Masdeu, J., O'Connel, R. *et al.* (1994) Brain perfusion abnormalities following minor/moderate closed head injury: comparison between early and late imaging in two groups of patients. *European Journal of Nuclear Medicine*, **21**, 750.

26. Gray, B.G., Ichise, M., Chung, D. *et al.* (1992) Technetium 99-m HMPAO SPECT in the evaluation of patient with a remote history of traumatic brain injury: a comparison with X-ray computed tomography. *Journal of Nuclear Medicine*, **33**, 52–58.

27. Silberstein, S., Lipton, R. and Goadsby, P. (1998) Post-traumatic headache, in *Headache in Clinical Practice* (eds S. Silberstein, R. Lipton and P. Goadsby), Oxford University Press, Corby, p. 140.

28. Weiss, H.D., Sterm, B.J. and Goldbert, J. (1991) Post traumatic migraine: chronic migraine precipitated by minor head or neck trauma. *Headache*, **31**, 451–456.

29. Haas, D.C. and Laurie, H. (1988) Trauma-triggered migraine: an explanation for common neurologic attacks after mild head injury. *Journal of Neurosurgery*, **68**, 181–188.

30. Jensen, O.K. and Nielsen, F.F. (1990) The influence of sex and pretraumatic headache on the incidence and severity of headache after head injury. *Cephalalgia: An International Journal of Headache*, **10**, 285–293.

31. Russell, M.B. and Olesen, J. (1996) Migraine associated with head trauma and its relation to migraine. *European Journal of Neurology*, **3**, 424–428.

32. Medina, J.L. (1992) Efficacy of an individualized outpatient program in the treatment of chronic post-traumatic headache. *Headache*, **32**, 180–183.

33. Packard, R.C. and Ham, L.P. (1993) Post-traumatic headache: determining chronicity. *Headache*, **33**, 133–134.

34. Packard, R.C. (1992) Post-traumatic headache: permanency and relationship to legal settlement. *Headache*, **32**, 496–504.

35. Kraus, J.F., Fife, D., Cox, P. *et al.* (1986) Incidence, severity and external causes of pediatric brain injury. *American Journal of Diseases of Children*, **140**, 687–693.

36. Silberstein, S., Lipton, R., Goadsby, P. (1998) Post-traumatic headache, in Headache in Clinical Practice (eds S. Silberstein, R. Lipton and P. Goadsby), Oxford University Press, Corby, p. 137.

37. Goldman, P.S. (1974) An alternative to development plasticity: heterology of CNS structures in infants and adults, in *Plasticity and Recovery from Brain Damage* (eds D.G. Stein, J.J. Rosen and N. Butters), Academic, Orlando, pp. 149–174.

38. Mahoney, W.J., D'Souza, B.J., Haller, J.A. *et al.* (1983) Long-term outcome of children with severe head trauma and prolonged coma. *Pediatrics*, **71**, 756–762.

39. Kriel, R.L., Krach, L.E. and Panser, L.A. (1989) Closed head injury: comparison of children younger and older than 6 years of age. *Pediatric Neurology*, **5**, 296–300.

40. Filley, C.M., Cranberg, I.D., Alexander, M.P. and Hart, E.J. (1987) Neurobehavioral outcome after closed head injury in childhood and adolescence. *Archives of Neurology*, **44**, 194–198.

41. Kolb, B. (1989) Brain development, plasticity, and behavior. *American Psychologist*, **44**, 1203–1212.

42. Ewing-Cobbs, L., Levin, H.S., Eisenberg, H.M. and Fletcher, J.M. (1987) Language functions following closed-head injury in children and adolescents. *Journal of Clinical and Experimental Neuropsychology*, **9**, 575–592.

43. Dikman, S., McLean, A. and Temkin, N. (1986) Neuropsychological and psychosocial consequences of minor head injury. *Journal of Neurology, Neurosurgery, and Psychiatry*, **49**, 1227–1232.

44. Fay, G.C., Jaffe, K.M., Polissar, N.L. *et al.* (1993) Mild pediatric traumatic brain injury: a cohort study. *Archives of Physical Medicine and Rehabilitation*, **74**, 895–901.

45. Denker, P.G. (1944) The postconcussion syndrome: prognosis and evaluation of the organic factors. *New York State Journal of Medicine*, **44**, 379–384.

46. Dencker, S.J. and Lofving, B.A. (1958) A psychometric study of identical twins discordant for closed head injury. *Acta Psychiatrica et Neurologica Scandinavica*, **122** (Suppl. 33), 1–50.

47. Rutherford, W.H., Merrett, J.D. and McDonald, J.R. (1977) Sequelae of concussion caused by minor head injuries. *Lancet*, **1**, 14.

48. Headache Classification Subcommittee of the International Headache (2004) The International Classification of Headache Disorders. *Cephalalgia: An International Journal of Headache*, **24** (Suppl 1), 1–160.

16
Headaches associated with altered intracranial pressure

Andrew D. Hershey

One form of secondary headache that can be seen in children is headaches associated with altered intracranial pressure. Two forms of altered intracranial pressure can occur, namely increased and decreased, with the more notably recognized being increased intracranial pressure. The most common reason for decreased intracranial pressure that results in headache is typically due to a persistent dural leak. The International Classification of Headache Disorders (ICHD)-II [1] identifies these two disorders together under headache attributed to nonvascular intracranial disorder. Increased intracranial pressure is described as headache attributed to high cerebral spinal fluid (CSF) pressure (ICHD-II, 7.1) whereas low cerebral spinal fluid pressure is described in ICHD-II 7.2. Increased intracranial pressure can be idiopathic or secondary to an underlying etiology, including metabolic, toxic or a mass effect with or without hydrocephalus. Low intracranial pressure, on the other hand, is typically due to a persistent loss of CSF, including either following lumbar puncture or due to a CSF fistula, trauma or spontaneous drop in intracranial pressure.

16.1 Increased intracranial pressure

Within the skull there are three major components: the brain, blood and CSF. This fixed space instituted by the skull means that an increase in any one of these components will result in pressure on the dura and subsequent irritation of the

Pediatric Headaches in Clinical Practice   Andrew D. Hershey, Paul Winner, Marielle A. Kabbouche and Scott W. Powers
© 2009 John Wiley & Sons, Ltd.

dural nerves (predominantly the first branch of the trigeminal nerve) and pain. For this to cause pain, the change in pressure needs to be acute or sub-acute, as the dura will adapt to a slow change in pressure or a mass such as is seen in a stable arachnoid cyst. An increase in brain mass is most associated with a tumor or a mass-type lesion and will be discussed in Chapter 17. Similarly, an increase in blood volume is either due to a mass such as an arterial venous malformation or large aneurysm, a leakage of the blood vessels such as subarachnoid hemorrhage, or due to increased arterial pressure that may be metabolic or chronic in nature. When there is an increase in CSF pressure without other underlying etiology, this is most often referred to as idiopathic intracranial hypertension (IIH).

Intracranial hypertension can be either idiopathic, without a clear etiology, or symptomatic of an underlying pathology. ICHD-II identifies the essential components of IIH (Table 16.1). By definition there is raised intracranial

Table 16.1 Headache attributed to IIH. (ICHD- II criteria reproduced with permission from Blackwell Publishing)

Previously used terms
Benign intracranial hypertension (BIH), pseudotumor cerebri, meningeal hydrops, serous meningitis.

Diagnostic criteria
A. Progressive headache with at least one of the following characteristics and fulfilling criteria C and D:
   1. Daily occurrence.
   2. Diffuse and/or constant (non-pulsating) pain.
   3. Aggravated by coughing or straining.
B. Intracranial hypertension fulfilling the following criteria:
   1. Alert patient with neurological examination that either is normal or demonstrates any of the following abnormalities:
      (a) papilledema
      (b) enlarged blind spot
      (c) visual field defect (progressive if untreated)
      (d) sixth nerve palsy.
   2. Increased CSF pressure (>200 mm H_2O in the nonobese, >250 mm H_2O in the obese) measured by lumbar puncture in the recumbent position or by epidural or intraventricular pressure monitoring.
   3. Normal CSF chemistry (low CSF protein is acceptable) and cellularity.
   4. Intracranial diseases (including venous sinus thrombosis) ruled out by appropriate investigations.
   5. No metabolic, toxic or hormonal cause of intracranial hypertension.
C. Headache develops in close temporal relation to increased intracranial pressure.
D. Headache improves after withdrawal of CSF to reduce pressure to 120–170 mm H_2O and resolves within 72 h of persistent normalization of intracranial pressure.

---

pressure with the absence of any other space-occupying or vascular lesions. Therefore, one of the essential steps in the identification of IIH is ruling out a space-occupying lesion. This relates to the former terms for IIH, including pseudo-tumor cerebri, where it appeared the patient had a tumor but no tumor was evident. The second essential component in the diagnosis once an intracranial lesion has been eliminated is elevated intracranial pressure. Some reviews have raised the possibility of normal pressure and only a moderate increase in pressure with similar symptomology. There may, therefore, be a spectrum within this disorder without any clearly defined limit as to when intracranial hypertension has elevated pressure by lumbar puncture.

Incidence

The incidence of intracranial hypertension is approximately 1 out of 100 000, with a range of reported studies from 0.9 to 2.2%. It appears to be more common in women and more common in obese individuals, although it does occur in men and does occur in nonobese individuals. The incidence in childhood is unclear, although it has been clearly observed.

Clinical characteristics

For headaches caused by IIH, there is a direct correspondence to increased intracranial pressure. ICHD-II establishes increased pressure as >200 mm CSF for nonobese individuals and >250 mm CSF for obese individuals. The headache associated with this increase for IIH is often daily.

The headache pain associated with IIH can be variable [2, 3]. Typically, the headache is described as moderate, is often chronic and may be progressive. It may start as episodic and progress to chronic over weeks. Oftentimes, the headache resembles migraine or tension-type headache and occasionally may have a pulsatile quality. Physical activity, including Valsalva and postural changes, can aggravate the pain.

Visual symptoms are often reported and can include seeing dark patches or spots. This can involve either one eye or both eyes. It can progress to visual loss that typically lasts less than a minute [4]. Evaluation of the retina can reveal the typical clinical sign in IIH: increased ocular pressure with papilledema. Classically, it is thought that papilledema is directly reflective on intracranial pressure. Papilledema has been integrally tied with IIH, although case reports do exist of IIH without papilledema.

In a study by of 25 consecutive patients with chronic daily headaches, increased opening pressure above 200 mm of CSF by lumbar punctures was found but no papilledema was evident [5]. Control patients consisted of chronic daily headache patients who had normal CSF. The two features that differentiated these groups were a pulsatile tinnitus in the patients with moderately elevated opening pressure and obesity. Of note, the opening pressure did vary from 200 to 550 mm of CSF for all patients that were diagnosed with the increased intracranial pressure without papilledema and had an opening pressure of at least 240 mm of CSF at some time during the study. This would suggest that, in patients with chronic daily headaches that had pulsatile tinnitus or obesity, a lumbar puncture should be considered to identify a possible increased IIH.

An alternative to measuring intracranial pressure when lumbar puncture is unavailable or contraindicated is measuring intraocular pressures. In a study of 50 patients who underwent lumbar puncture, CSF pressure and intraocular pressure was measured simultaneously [6]. There was very close agreement between intraocular pressure and CSF pressure as measured by lumbar puncture. As this procedure is less invasive, it may serve as a method to supplant and identify increased intracranial hypertension.

Once an increase in intracranial pressure has been identified, other etiologies need to be ruled out. These etiologies can include medications, both prescribed and nonprescribed, for a variety of conditions and endocrinologic etiologies (Table 16.2). One underlying pathophysiological contribution that appears to be related to these etiologies is fat solubility. One of the compounds that have been suspected to contribute to increased intracranial hypertension is vitamin A, either from excessive dietary intake or from prescriptions. In children, this may be the case in the treatment of acne and can also include retinoids with an elevation of vitamin A or vitamin A-like compounds. If an elevated vitamin A level is suspected, then the level should be measured and the etiology of this elevation investigated.

Some medications, including antibiotics used to treat acne in adolescents (e.g. tetracycline, minocycline and doxycycline), have been noted to be associated with an increased risk of IIH. The association of IIH with obesity may be due to contributions from obesity-related conditions, including hypertension or possible polycystic ovary disease. In women, there has also been an association with pregnancy, as well as with hormonal therapy and menstrual dysfunction.

Pathophysiology

Several pathophysiological models exist to explain intracranial hypertension. At the basis of this disorder is the recognition that the skull contains CSF, brain and blood; therefore, elevation or a swelling of any of these components may contribute to intracranial hypertension.

Table 16.2 Potential causes of increased intracranial pressure. (ICHD-II criteria reproduced with permission from Blackwell Publishing)

Anatomical lesion
Tumor
Vascular lesion
Chiari malformation
Turner syndrome

Endocrine
Pituitary/adrenal
    Cushing's disease
    Corticosteroid therapy or withdrawal
    Addison's disease
Thyroid disease (hyper or hypo)
Parathyroid disease
Obesity
Polycystic ovary syndrome

Hematologic
Anemia
Polycythemia
Coagulation disorders

Infectious
Chronic encephalitis/meningitis
HIV
Lyme disease

Medications
Vitamin A and related compounds, including isotretinoin, *all-trans*-retionic acid
Antibiotics (tetracycline, nalidixic acid, nitrofurantoin, sulfonamides)
NSAIDs (indomethacin, refecoxib)
Cyclosporine
Lithium
Cimetidine

Vascular
Venous sinus thrombosis

Increased CSF volume

Increased CSF production is rare but has been noted in choroid plexus papilloma, a disorder of childhood. Decreased CSF absorption has been speculated based on reports of decreased CSF circulation during isotopic cysternograms. It has been theorized that there may be a blockage of CSF resorption in the arachnoid granules. This is currently hypothetical, but may explain the increase in intracranial pressure associated with meningoencephalitis or other disorders of increased CSF viscosity in which the arachnoid granules are unable to resorb CSF effectively.

Increased brain volume

There has been a suggestion that increased water deposition in the brain may contribute to intracranial hypertension, based on selected MRI studies; however, the number is small and the variation is limited. This does occur in edema of the brain following an ischemic lesion or traumatic injury, but this should be differentiated as a post-vascular or posttraumatic headache and identifiable by MRI or neuroimaging. Fat solubility of compounds may also account for increased brain volume. It has been observed that fat-soluble vitamins and fat-soluble compounds are associated with increased intracranial hypertension. Although no clear cause and effect has been observed, it could be speculated that dissolution of fat-soluble compounds within the brain could cause increased brain volume and subsequently cause enough increased pressure to contribute to increased intracranial hypertension.

Increased vascular volume

This can be due to a vascular lesion, an increase in arterial flow or a decrease in venous drainage. A vascular lesion would be eliminated as a cause by neuroimaging. An increase in arterial pressure is less likely to contribute to IIH, but may be a consequence of lost autoregulation following an ischemic or traumatic insult.

A blockage of venous drainage has been demonstrated to occur in several models of IIP and may explain the common convergence of multiple etiologies. Venograms have shown narrowing of cerebral veins suggestive of blocked outflow. In a study of 29 patients compared with 59 control patients using magnetic resonance venograms, it was found that 27 of the 29 patients had an increase in intracranial pressure compared with 4 of the 59 controls [7]. These patients had bilateral sinovenous stenosis, suggesting that the stenosis of these blood vessels, and therefore lack of venous drainage, may be a contributor to the pathology of IIH.

In a study of 21 patients that clinically had IIH with headache and papilledema by using manometry combined with cervical puncture, it was found that venous hypertension was present and that the venous hypertension resolved after C1, C2 puncture [8]. The source of the hypertension appeared to be compression of venous outflow at the transverse sinus with a marked drop in pressure distal from this point. This compression of the transverse sinus resulted in increased intracranial pressure; once the pressure is relieved, the venous sinus pressure returned to normal. This is suggestive of a feedback phenomenon in which the increased intracranial hypertension contributes to the transverse sinus compression and, therefore, contributes to increased intracranial hypertension in a feedback loop. Once the pressure has dropped and the transverse sinus is able to return to normal flow, the CSF pressure can also return to normal flow. This observation raises further questions as to what is the etiological factor that starts this event. It does appear that venous obstruction or contribution to venous obstruction augments the fact of IIH.

Treatment

Medical management

Once it is determined that the IIH is not secondary to another underlying cause, treatment needs to be initiated. As discussed above, there may be a feedback loop established that can be broken by lowering the intracranial pressure. Therefore, it is expected that patients will have an improvement or resolution of their headache following a lumbar puncture. When performing a lumbar puncture, assurance must be made to note the reduction of CSF pressure into the normal range. Repeated lumbar puncture may allow for a draining of this fluid to allow for returning to normal pressure. If this is unsuccessful or undesirable due to repeat of lumbar punctures, other management can include medical management, weight reduction and surgical management. Medical management consists predominantly of lowering CSF production. This can be done through carbonic anhydrase inhibitors (acetazolamide, topiramate) or through diuretics. No controlled studies have shown overall effectiveness of combining carbonic anhydrase inhibitors, diuretics or, in rare instances, cortical steroids.

Weight reduction has been noted to have resolution of papilledema and headaches, including possible surgical intervention to assist with weight reduction.

Surgical management

If medical management and weight reduction are not successful and if visual changes have been noted, then surgical management is warranted. The role of surgical management is to lower CSF pressure and preserve visual function.

This surgical treatment can include shunting, either a ventricle peritoneal or lumbar peritoneal shunt. However, the success rate for increased intracranial hypertension is low. Alternative optic nerve sheath fenestration has been demonstrated to allow for decompression of the optic nerve. It appears that this may allow CSF leakage as well as preserve compression on the optic nerve and, therefore, assist with visual perseveration.

Based on the potential etiology of IIH by venous stenosis, stenting of the venous sinuses has been suggested as a treatment in chronic, refractory patients with IIH [9]. In a study of 10 patients, six patients were asymptomatic following stenting, with all patients' papilledema resolving. This intervention provides potential long-term improvement in patients that are refractory to medical or other surgical treatment.

Outcomes

Historically, it has been reported that the outcome of IIH is a return to normal function. In a study of 410 patients diagnosed with IIH seen from 1984 to 1996, there were 20 patients followed over a 10-year period [10]. Of the 20 patients, 11 patients were stable without changes in visual field of papilledema while nine patients had a worsening after a stable course. From this very limited study, this suggests that IIH may have a chronic component and may not be just a single event; therefore, long-term management and observation may be necessary.

16.2 Decreased intracranial pressure

Headaches can also be caused by low CSF pressure (for review, see Mokri [11]). The most typical example of this is a post-lumbar-puncture headache. Historically, this was first noted by Quincke in 1891 and first recorded by Bier in 1898. By 1938 it was recognized that spontaneous decreased CSF pressure could also be noted. The typical clinical presentation of a post-lumbar headache is a headache worsening with positioning, especially standing, after a lumbar puncture or a procedure in which the dura is disrupted.

ICHD-II has established criteria for the diagnosis of CSF hypotension headaches (Table 16.3). Three broad categories of headache attributed to low CSF pressure were detailed: post-dural/post-lumbar puncture headache; CSF fistula headache; and headache attributed to spontaneous or idiopathic low CSF pressure. The diagnostic criteria for all three types require resolution of the headache pain after closure of the CSF leak and return of pressure to normal.

Table 16.3   Headache attributed to low CSF pressure

7.2.1 Post-dural (post-lumbar) puncture headache
Diagnostic criteria
A. Headache that worsens within 15 min after sitting or standing and improves within 15 min after lying, with at least one of the following and fulfilling criteria C and D:
1. Neck stiffness.
2. Tinnitus.
3. Hypacusia.
4. Photophobia.
5. Nausea.
B. Dural puncture has been performed.
C. Headache develops within 5 days after dural puncture.
D. Headache resolves either:
1. Spontaneously within 1 week.
2. Within 48 h after effective treatment of the spinal fluid leak (usually by epidural blood patch).

7.2.2 CSF fistula headache
Diagnostic criteria
A. Headache that worsens within 15 min after sitting or standing, with at least one of the following and fulfilling criteria C and D:
1. Neck stiffness.
2. Tinnitus.
3. Hypacusia.
4. Photophobia.
5. Nausea.
B. A known procedure or trauma has caused persistent CSF leakage with at least one of the following:
1. Evidence of low CSF pressure on MRI (e.g. pachymeningeal enhancement).
2. Evidence of CSF leakage on conventional myelography, CT myelography or cisternography.
3. CSF opening pressure <60 mm H_2O in sitting position.
C. Headache develops in close temporal relation to CSF leakage.
D. Headache resolves within 7 days of sealing the CSF leak.

7.2.3 Headache attributed to spontaneous (or idiopathic) low CSF pressure
Previously used terms
Spontaneous intracranial hypotension, primary intracranial hypotension, low CSF-volume headache, hypoliquorrheic headache.

Diagnostic criteria
A. Diffuse and/or dull headache that worsens within 15 min after sitting or standing, with at least one of the following and fulfilling criterion D:
1. Neck stiffness.
2. Tinnitus.
3. Hypacusia.

Table 16.3 (*Continued*)

---

    4. Photophobia.

    5. Nausea.

B. At least one of the following:

    1. Evidence of low CSF pressure on MRI (e.g. pachymeningeal enhancement).

    2. Evidence of CSF leakage on conventional myelography, CT myelography or cisternography.

    3. CSF opening pressure <60 mm H_2O in sitting position.

C. No history of dural puncture or other cause of CSF fistula.

D. Headache resolves within 72 h after epidural blood patching.

Clinical features

As can be noted from ICHD-II, the clinical features of the headache are common for all three syndromes and includes a postural headache that worsens with sitting or standing and improves by lying down. These headaches may have a throbbing quality, but can vary by position and activity. The headache location is typically frontal but may be holocephalic or nuchal. It is typically bilateral and may evolve into a chronic daily headache. The pain may worsen as the day progresses, especially in sustained upright positions, and be relieved by lying down overnight. Typical associated symptoms include neck stiffness, tinnitus, hypacusia, photophobia and nausea. Other clinical symptoms may include horizontal diplopia, cranial nerve palsies (CN III and VI), visual and hearing changes, and may progress to encephalopathic signs [11].

The orthostatic nature of these headaches has raised the potential of using positioning as a diagnostic tool. Rozen *et al.* [12] found that patients in the Trendelenburg position with a CSF leak may have resolution of their headaches.

When performing a lumbar puncture, CSF pressure should be low, but may also be a 'dry tap' with normal to increased protein and normal glucose. An MRI scan may have pachymeningeal enhancement with subdural collections and some evidence of the brain sagging. Additional MRI findings include enlargement of the pituitary and engorgement of the venous signs and decreased size of the ventricles. As the investigation into the location of the CSF leakage persists, spinal MRI may identify a leak at the cervical–thoracic junction, although this is oftentimes very difficult to identify. Radioisotope cisternography may also assist in identifying where the leakage occurs. Other studies include CT myography, including both fast flow and slow flow to identify where the leakage is.

Pathophysiology

The initial pathophysiology was thought to be due to a low pressure due to CSF leakage. It was speculated that this was due to a lag in CSF production compared with CSF leakage. With the advance of MRI studies and the observation of pachymeningeal enhancement with gadolinium in this group of patients [13], it appears that the underlying etiology of the pain and neurological symptoms is due to brain sag that resolves when the brain is allowed to float back into proper position, either by correcting the leak or loss of CSF fluid or in the recumbent or Trendelenburg position. Additional MRI findings included subdural fluid collections and descent of the cerebellar tonsils mimicking a Chiari I with a decreased size of the pre-pontine and fairly charismatic cisterns, flattening of the optic chiasma and crowding of the posterior fossa. This brain sagging appears to pull on the dura connections, causing dura irritation, and may explain the underlying etiology from the low CSF pressure not allowing the brain to float; therefore, having the patient lie recumbent relieves this pressure, as well as relieving the headaches.

Treatment

Treatment of low CSF pressure headaches includes bed rest, to relieve the pain, and hydration. It has been suggested that caffeine, administration either oral or intravenous, may assist with closure of the CSF leak, especially after a post-lumbar headache. If this is not successful, then an epidural patch may be required. This can include a blood patch using the patient's own blood. In addition, surgical glue has been reported to be useful in assisting with closing the hole once one it is identified. None of these treatments has been on controlled studies to identify their overall effectiveness, and oftentimes the search for the underlying CSF leak can be very difficult.

References

1. Headache Classification Subcommittee of the International Headache Society (2004) The International Classification of Headache Disorders. *Cephalagia*, **24** (Suppl. 1), 1–160.
2. Skau, M., Brennum, J., Gjerris, F. and Jensen, R. (2006) What is new about idiopathic intracranial hypertension? An updated review of mechanism and treatment. *Cephalalgia: An International Journal of Headache*, **26**(4), 384–399.
3. Ball, A.K. and Clarke, C.E. (2006) Idiopathic intracranial hypertension. *Lancet Neurology*, **5**(5), 433–442.

4. Wall, M. and George, D. (1991) Idiopathic intracranial hypertension. A prospective study of 50 patients. *Brain: A Journal of Neurology*, **114**(Pt 1A), 155–180.

5. Wang, S.J., Silberstein, S.D., Patterson, S. and Young, W. (1998) Idiopathic intracranial hypertension without papilledema: a case–control study in a headache center. *Neurology*, **51**, 245–249.

6. Sajjadi, S.A., Harirchian, M.H., Sheikhbahaei, N. *et al.* (2006) The relation between intracranial and intraocular pressures: study of 50 patients. *Annals of Neurology*, **59** (5), 867–870.

7. Farb, R.I., Vanek, I., Scott, J.N. *et al.* (2003) Idiopathic intracranial hypertension: the prevalence and morphology of sinovenous stenosis. *Neurology*, **60**(9), 1418–1424.

8. King, J.O., Mitchell, P.J., Thomson, K.R. and Tress, B.M. (2002) Manometry combined with cervical puncture in idiopathic intracranial hypertension. *Neurology*, **58**(1), 26–30.

9. Donnet, A., Metellus, P., Levrier, O. *et al.* (2008) Endovascular treatment of idiopathic intracranial hypertension: clinical and radiologic outcome of 10 consecutive patients. *Neurology*, **70** (8), 641–647.

10. Shah, V.A., Kardon, R.H., Lee, A.G. *et al.* (2008) Long-term follow-up of idiopathic intracranial hypertension: the Iowa experience. *Neurology*, **70**(8), 634–640.

11. Mokri, B. (2004) Low cerebrospinal fluid pressure syndromes. *Neurologic Clinics*, **22** (1), 55–74.

12. Rozen, T., Swidan, S., Hamel, P.-C. and Saper, J. (2008) Trendelenburg position: a tool to screen for the presence of a low CSF pressure syndrome in daily headache patients. *Headache*, in press 10.1111/j.15264610.2007.01027.x.

13. Mokri, B., Piepgras, D.G., Miller, G.M. (1997) Syndrome of orthostatic headaches and diffuse pachymeningeal gadolinium enhancement. *Mayo Clinic Proceedings*, **72** (5), 400–413.

17

Other secondary headaches

Andrew D. Hershey

As discussed throughout this text, headaches can be designated as primary or secondary headaches. Primary headaches are defined by their clinical features with specific, although overlapping features. One of the keys to the diagnosis of primary headaches is the lack of an identifiable etiology after a thorough history, physical examination and neurological examination of a secondary cause. When a secondary cause is suspected, then an investigation into the contribution of this component must be investigated to identify secondary headaches and, therefore, to begin the appropriate treatment if available for this secondary cause. Consequently, a confirmation of the diagnosis of a secondary headache is only available after successful treatment of the underlying etiology; and when this does not happen, a further investigation is warranted.

Secondary headaches by definition are headaches in which an underlying disorder initiates and perpetuates the headache. The International Classification of Headache Disorders (ICHD)-II criteria [1] change this relationship for 'associated with' to 'attributed to'. This somewhat subtle change highlights the importance of a direct cause and effect relationship of the headache due to the secondary cause. Secondary headaches have a cause and effect relationship and, thus, are less likely to be recurrent; but when they are recurrent, this implies that either the underlying etiology has not been successfully managed or that the diagnosis is inaccurate. This lack of recurrent nature and inaccuracy of

Pediatric Headaches in Clinical Practice   Andrew D. Hershey, Paul Winner, Marielle A. Kabbouche and Scott W. Powers
© 2009 John Wiley & Sons, Ltd.

diagnosis makes the study of secondary headaches difficult, with only a few generalizing principles. The simplest principles are:

1. Identification of a known cause of secondary headaches either by history or laboratory testing/neuroimaging.

2. Temporal and causal relationship between the identified disorder and the headache.

3. With adequate, effective treatment the headache resolves or is greatly reduced in an expected time course of the treatment or spontaneous resolution.

4. Unless the secondary cause is episodic, then episodic headaches are typically primary. If the secondary cause is episodic, then all of the other features of the secondary headache should also be present (i.e. temporal relation, response to treatment).

5. Patients with primary headaches can also get secondary headaches.

Some of the various etiologic categories causing secondary headaches are listed in ICDH-II (Table 17.1). Some of these secondary headaches have been discussed in previous chapters (sinus headaches in Chapter 14, posttraumatic headaches in Chapter 15, and headaches attributed to changes in intracranial pressure in Chapter 16), while medication-overuse headaches are addressed in several of the chapters on migraine, chronic migraine and treatment of primary headaches. Additional causes of secondary headaches that raise concern include headaches due to underlying metabolic disturbances, headaches due to intracranial masses (including brain tumors or vascular malformations) and headaches due to particular substances and their withdrawal.

17.1 Epidemiology

The prevalence of secondary headache varies considerably, depending upon specialty practice and the location of the evaluation. The lack of recurrence of secondary headaches, once successful treatment is employed, makes the identification of secondary headaches in a population-based study difficult. One exception is with headaches attributed to sinus disease (Chapter 14). This is due

Table 17.1 Secondary headaches [1]. (ICHD-II criteria reproduced with permission from Blackwell Publishing)

Head or neck trauma (Chapter 15)	ICHD-II, 5
Acute post-traumatic	ICHD-II, 5.1
Chronic post-traumatic	ICHD-II, 5.2
Vascular disorders	ICHD-II, 6
Ischemic stroke or TIA	ICHD-II, 6.1
Nontraumatic intracranial hemorrhage	ICHD-II, 6.2
Unruptured vascular malformation	ICHD-II, 6.3
Intracranial vascular disorder	ICHD-II, 6.7
Intracranial abnormalities, nonvascular	ICHD-II, 7
High pressure-CSF (Chapter 16)	ICHD-II, 7.1
Low pressure-CSF (Chapter 16)	ICHD-II, 7.2
Non-infection CNS inflammation	ICHD-II, 7.3
Neoplasm	ICHD-II, 7.4
Seizure related	ICHD-II, 7.6
Chiari malformation	ICHD-II, 7.7
Substances or their withdrawal	ICHD-II, 8.0
Acute exposure or use	ICHD-II, 8.1
Medication overuse	ICHD-II, 8.2
Substance withdrawal	ICHD-II, 8.4
Infection	ICHD-II, 9
Intracranial	ICHD-II, 9.1
Systemic	ICHD-II, 9.2
Metabolic/Homeostatic Disorders	ICHD-II, 10
Disorders of	
Cranium	ICHD-II, 11.1
Neck	ICHD-II, 11.2
Eyes	ICHD-II, 11.3
Ears	ICHD-II, 11.4
Rhinosinusitis (Chapter 14)	ICHD-II, 11.5
Teeth, jaw	ICHD-II, 11.6
TMJ	ICHD-II, 11.7
Psychiatric disorders	ICHD-II, 12
Cranial Neuralgias	ICHD-II, 13

to the episodic nature of sinus disease and allergies. This has led to much confusion in the diagnosis of sinus headache, with many of these patients actually having migraine and recurrent allergies as two separate conditions.

The overwhelming percentage of children and adolescents evaluated in the primary care physician's office with a recurrent complaint of headache have a primary headache such as migraine or tension-type headache (TTH). When a secondary headache presents, the parents typically have a very clear onsetting event. The secondary headache is typically a nonlife-threatening underlying medical or neurologic disorder. In patients with recurrent headaches, the secondary headache is often notably different, although there can be variation in primary headaches. Most commonly, this secondary headache is due to viral systemic infection, such as the 'flu' or secondary to otitis media or pharyngitis [2, 3].

In the emergency department, a secondary headache has an increased likelihood of an underlying neurologic disorder or medical disorder with neurological complications [4–6] – although the most frequent etiology remains a primary headache or mild infection (Chapter 6). Approximately 6–10% of children and adolescents seen in the emergency department will have an underlying systemic or neurologic disorder. If the patient has an underlying medical disorder, fever or trauma, then a secondary etiology to the headache should be sought. A thorough history and physical and neurological examinations will, in most cases, uncover the etiology and determine the need for a more in-depth evaluation (Chapter 2).

17.2 Evaluation

The medical model for the evaluation of headaches includes a thorough history. Parameters for the evaluation of a child presenting with headache have been published, with several caveats in the evaluation noted [7]. One key component in the evaluation is the physician's clinical index of suspicion when things do not seem right. In the case of secondary headaches, special attention must be given to 'red flags', including:

1. Symptoms of increased intracranial pressure.

2. Abrupt change in headache pattern, including recent onset or change in severity, frequency or associated symptoms.

3. First headache or worst headache ever.

4. Systemic symptoms or signs, especially of cerebrospinal fluid (CSF) infection or alterations of mental status.

5. A clear triggering event by recent history (i.e. trauma).

6. Early morning headache or headache that awakens from sleep.

Patients with a pre-existing medical disorder may have increased risk of developing a secondary headache with other systemic symptoms, such as fever, or symptoms of increased intracranial pressure. The headache history needs to include both the acute cause and effect relationship when a secondary headache is suspected, but also needs to include a review of other symptoms and past medical history of suspected disorders. A family history of recurrent headaches can be reassuring of a primary headache disorder, but is only one component in the evaluation for secondary headaches.

The physical examination begins with a thorough general pediatric examination and is followed by a neurologic examination and comprehensive headache examination (see Chapter 2). Attention should be paid to any evidence of altered vital signs, trauma, meningismus and rash. Papilledema, extraocular movements, asymmetric reflexes or weakness, ataxia and dysmetria should be noted. The patient's mental status should be carefully evaluated. Based on this history and examination, additional testing may be warranted (Chapter 3).

After a complete history and examinations, a clear concept of the headaches being either primary or secondary should be evident; if not, then additional history, testing or observation may be necessary. Oftentimes, clinical experience and a high index of suspicion when the evaluation seems unusual allow the physician to differentiate between a sick child needing further evaluation immediately and an otherwise well child with a significant but nonlife-threatening headache. The presence of abnormal neurologic symptoms, progressive headache or abnormal neurological examination mandates the need for further evaluation.

Deciding on whether or not an imaging procedure is needed is difficult and cannot always be based on guidelines [7]. Once again, if it is not clear as to the etiology or there is a question to the etiology and 'red flags' are present, neuroimaging may be important to eliminate a life-threatening or potentially treatable cause. It should be noted that abnormalities seen in the scan do not always account for the patient's symptoms [8].

Headaches are a common complaint seen by the primary care practitioners. It is the fifth most common disorder seen in the primary care physician's office and follows allergy, otitis media, asthma and eczema. Therefore, differentiating primary headaches from secondary headaches is essential. Primary headaches are usually recurrent and typically not associated with life-threatening disorders [2, 3]. In one series, children in a primary care office with headache often had noncentral nervous infections. Infectious disorders were important in 22 of 37 patients and included viral infections, pharyngitis, otitis and sinusitis [3]. Patients with headache have an increased incidence of sleep disorders, and individuals with sleep problems have an increased incidence of headache [9, 10]. Headaches secondary to mild head trauma without neurologic symptoms or signs are also common, as are headaches secondary to medication and substance abuse. It should be emphasized that ocular disorders and serious medical or neurological problems are uncommon in the otherwise well child.

Several studies have been published looking at the frequency, etiology and evaluation of headaches in children and adolescents presenting to the emergency department (reviewed in Chapter 6). Approximately 5–7% of all children presenting to the emergency room have the chief complaint of headache. These children may have the acute onset of a primary or secondary headache, an acute attack of a recurrent headache or progression of a chronic headache. Of children seen in emergency departments, anywhere from 2 to 15% have a serious underlying medical or neurological problem as the etiology of their headaches. The remainder of conditions includes stress-related headaches, migraine headaches and headaches associated with infectious disorders or mild trauma. The etiology of significant neurologic or medical conditions includes hydrocephalus, shunt malfunction, aseptic meningitis, bacterial meningitis, brain abscess, substance abuse, trauma, metabolic dysfunction, neoplasms and vascular disorders.

17.3 Selected secondary headaches

Several of the most common etiologies of secondary headaches are directly addressed in other chapters. A thorough review of secondary headaches can be *The Headaches*, third edition [11] or *Wolff's Headaches and Other Head Pain*, eighth edition [12]. The remainder of this chapter will highlight a few secondary headaches that can be seen in children.

Medical-systemic causes of headache

Secondary headaches can occur as a symptom of other medical problems or of primary neurologic disorders. This can include infections, metabolic disorders, renal problems, mitochondrial disorders, increased blood pressure and hematologic disorders. When a patient has a known medical condition, either the condition itself or the treatment may induce headaches. It must be kept in mind that patients with known medical problems are not protected from primary headaches, and if there is not a direct cause and effect and variation with treatment, then a diagnosis and management of a primary headache disorder should be considered.

Vascular disorders (ICHD-II, 6)

Vascular disorders can frequently have a headache as one of their symptoms [13]. This can be attributed to ischemia, hemorrhage or diseases of the blood vessels, including malformations, arteritis, injury to the vessels (i.e. dissection or surgical intervention), thrombosis or genetic diseases of the blood vessels (i.e. CADASIL, MELAS). These disorders for the most part are rare in children, but should be considered when other symptoms are present.

Cerebrovascular disease in children is rare, occurring at a rate of 2.5/100 000. Symptoms of acute neurological changes occur at the same time as the headache. This needs to be considered on the first presentation of hemiplegic migraine, even in the setting of a family history.

Hemorrhage may be secondary to rupture of a vascular malformation or aneurysm or secondary to trauma. The presenting symptom is most often an acute severe headache ('worst headache of my life') associated with loss of consciousness, meningismus and local neurologic symptoms. An underlying neurocutaneous disorder should be sought. If this diagnosis is suspected, then imaging will usually show the hemorrhage. Angiography or venography may delineate the specific etiology.

Vasculitis is being reported with increased frequency in children and adolescents, but remains uncommon. Headaches occur in 40–70% of patients with primary CNS vasculitis. It may occur in the setting of an autoimmune disorder, such as systemic lupus erythematosus, polyarteritis, Wegner's granulomatosis and Sjögren's syndrome. Although headaches may uncommonly be the initial symptom, other systemic symptoms have usually preceded the headache. The headaches may resemble either chronic TTH or migraine and usually exacerbate when the underlying autoimmune disorder worsens. Other neurologic symptoms may include behavioral changes, cognitive dysfunction, seizures and focal deficits. Magnetic resonance imaging (MRI) and magnetic resonance angiography may show abnormalities. CSF may be abnormal. Angiography may be required.

Emboli and thromboses may be idiopathic or secondary trauma, coagulation disorders, autoimmune disorders and congenital heart disease. Conditions such as moyamoya disease, fibromuscular dysplasia, arterial dissection, tumor, trauma, sickle cell anemia, hemophilia and dehydration may also cause secondary vascular disease.

Venous sinus thrombosis may occur in the presence of an underlying metabolic or systemic infection, a coagulation disorder or patients who are dehydrated. The patients may present with headache, altered consciousness, lethargy, focal neurologic symptoms and seizures. The neurologic examination is usually abnormal and the MRI scan, as well as magnetic resonance venography, may show the thrombosed vessel and/or hemorrhage secondary to venous thrombosis. Consideration should be given to this diagnosis in the presence of a coagulopathy, systemic malignancy and/or chemotherapy.

Neoplasms (ICHD-II, 7.4)

Intracranial tumors are the second most common type of neoplasm in children [14, 15]. In children younger than 15 years, the incidence is 2.4/100 000. Certain genetic syndromes, such as neurofibromatosis, tuberous sclerosis, von Hippel–Lindau diseases and ataxia telangiectasis, pose a greater risk for the development of neoplasms.

The fear of a brain tumor is one of the major concerns of parents bringing their children to the physician for evaluation of headache. However, the prevalence of primary headaches far outweighs the frequency of tumor-related headaches. There is a clear association between brain tumors and headaches, with the majority of brain tumors having headache as one of the presenting manifestations.

The headache due to a brain tumor is the result of increased intracranial pressure due to the mass effect of the tumor or a blockage of CSF drainage. In addition, the effects of the brain tumor on the surrounding tissue also induce changes in the neurological examination or neurological symptoms [7]. Other symptoms of brain tumor include seizures, ataxia, weakness, visual abnormalities, lethargy and personality change in the majority of such patients; the course will be progressive. The neurologic examination will be abnormal and the diagnosis can be confirmed by neuroimaging.

Owing to the continued growth of the tumor, the headache pattern is usually chronic, progressive with increases in frequency and severity over time. The rapidity of the growth of the tumor and the adaptability of the intracranial space to respond to this growth can modify the timing of the headache's presentation. Frequently, it is reported to occur in the morning due to a 'ball-valve' effect in which the CSF pressure builds in the recumbent position and is relieved by posture – the opposite of idiopathic intracranial hypertension (Chapter 16). If there is hemorrhage into the tumor, then the headache may also present more acutely.

Substance-induced headache (ICHD-II, 8)

Prescribed medications, illicit drugs, dietary compounds and toxins can cause headaches [16]. These substances may initiate a headache, exacerbate a pre-existing headache or cause headache on its withdrawal. A through history of exposure to medications and nonmedication needs to be performed, and removal or alteration of these substance, if possible, may be necessary before the headache responds. Stimulants used in the treatment of attention-deficit disorder may initiate headache, especially if they are restarted at maximum dosage after not having been taken for several days to weeks. One common stimulant used in children and adults is caffeine, and caffeine addiction and its withdrawal can contribute to headache and exacerbate primary headaches.

Medication-overuse headache (MOH) can occur with overuse of over-the-counter analgesic medication or prescription medications. This has formally been referred to as analgesic rebound headache. It is often associated with a gradual increase in frequency of medications that were successful or partially successful in headache treatment. These medications are typically taken at low doses or with repeated doses, building to very frequent usage – up to daily. By ICHD-II, using prescription medications more than 10 times per month or over-the-counter analgesics more than 15 times per month increase the likelihood of MOH. Almost all medications used for the acute treatment of migraine can potentially cause MOH. If MOH is thought to be a contributor to the development of frequent headaches, then they should be limited for 4–6 weeks. At that point they can be reintroduced, but at a limited frequency.

Infectious disorders (ICHD-II, 9)

Systemic infectious disorders or those localized to the central nervous system are commonly associated with headache. The presence of an elevated temperature and tachycardia alone frequently give rise to a pounding headache which is often relieved when the temperature is lowered and the infection is treated. Among the common infections seen are sinusitis, otitis media and pharyngitis. Among the infections affecting the central nervous system are meningitis, aseptic meningitis and encephalitis [17]. Brain abscess is uncommon. It occurs more commonly in children with cyanotic congenital heart disease, open head trauma, chronic ear infections, chronic pulmonary disease, post-neurosurgical procedures and in the immunocompromised patient.

In any central nervous system infection, in addition to symptoms of increased intracranial pressure or progressive neurologic disease, meningismus, rash or elevated temperature may be present. Initial evaluation should include a brain imaging procedure to rule out a mass lesion. If at all possible, this should be performed prior to any lumbar puncture.

17.4 Conclusions

The majority of recurrent headaches in children and adolescents are primary headaches. Secondary headaches, however, occur due to systemic or central nervous system disease. The history and physical examination should help identify this possibility, with appropriate laboratory tests and neuroimaging confirming the suspicion. Ultimately, the diagnosis of the secondary headache will be the resolution of the headache once the secondary cause has been effectively treated.

References

1. Headache Classification Subcommittee of the International Headache Society (2004) The International Classification of Headache Disorders. *Cephalagia*, **24** (Suppl. 1), 1–160.
2. Mortimer, M.J., Kay, J. and Jaron, A. (1992) Epidemiology of headache and childhood migraine in an urban general practice using ad hoc, Vahlquist and IHS criteria. *Developmental Medicine and Child Neurology*, **34**, 1095–1101.
3. Kandt, R.S. and Levine, R.M.(Jan 1987) Headache and acute illness in children. *Journal of Child Neurology*, **2**(1), 22–27.
4. Burton, L.J., Quinn, B., Pratt-Cheney, J.L. and Pourani, M. (1997) Headache etiology in a pediatric emergency department. *Pediatric Emergency Care*, **13**(1), 1–4.
5. Lewis, D.W. and Qureshi, F. (2000) Acute headache in children and adolescents presenting to the emergency department. *Headache*, **40**(3), 200–203.
6. Kabbouche, M.A. and Linder, S.L. (2005) Management of migraine in children and adolescents in the emergency department and inpatient setting. *Current Pain and Headache Reports*, **9**(5), 363–367.
7. Lewis, D.W., Ashwal, S., Dahl, G. *et al.* (2002) Practice parameter: evaluation of children and adolescents with recurrent headaches: report of the Quality Standards Subcommittee of the American Academy of Neurology and the Practice Committee of the Child Neurology Society. *Neurology*, **59**(4), 490–498.
8. Schwedt, T.J., Guo, Y. and Rothner, A.D. (2006) 'Benign' imaging abnormalities in children and adolescents with headache. *Headache*, **46**(3), 387–398.
9. Bruni, O., Febrizi, P., Ottaviano, S. *et al.* (1997) Prevalence of sleep disorders in childhood and adolescence with headache: a case–control study. *Cephalalgia: An International Journal of Headache*, **17**, 492–498.

10. Miller, V.A., Palermo, T.M., Powers, S.W. *et al.* (2003) Migraine headaches and sleep disturbances in children. *Headache*, **43**(4), 362–368.

11. Olesen, J., Goadsby, P., Ramadan, N. *et al.* (2006) *The Headaches*, 3rd edn, Lippincott, Williams & Wilkins, Philadelphia, PA.

12. Silberstein, S., Lipton, R. and Dodick, D. (2008) *Wolff's Headaches and Other Head Pain*, 8th edn, Oxford University Press, Inc., New York, NY.

13. Roach, E. and Riela, A. (1995) *Pediatric Cerebrovascular Disorders*, 2nd edn, Futura, New York.

14. The Childhood Brain Tumor Consortium (1991) The epidemiology of headache among children with brain tumor. Headache in children with brain tumors. *Journal of Neuro-Oncology*, **10**(1) 31–46.

15. Honig, P.J. and Charney, E.B. (1982) Children with brain tumor headaches. Distinguishing features. *American Journal of Diseases of Children*, **136**(2), 121–124.

16. Silberstein, S.D., Lipton, R.B. and Goadsby, P.J. (1998) *Headache in Clinical Practice*, Isis Medical Media, Ltd, Oxford, UK.

17. Bale, J.F. Jr. (1999) Human herpesviruses and neurological disorders of childhood. *Seminars in Pediatric Neurology*, **6**(4), 278–287.

Index

Note: page numbers in *italics* refer to figures and tables

Pediatric Headaches in Clinical Practice   Andrew D. Hershey, Paul Winner, Marielle A. Kabbouche and Scott W. Powers
© 2009 John Wiley & Sons, Ltd.

Index compiled by Jill Halliday